Nursing and Multi-professional Practice

Nursing and Multi-professional Practice

Edited by
Janet McCray

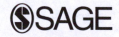

Los Angeles • London • New Delhi • Singapore • Washington DC

First published 2009

SAGE Publications Ltd
1 Oliver's Yard
55 City Road
London EC1Y 1SP

SAGE Publications Inc.
2455 Teller Road
Thousand Oaks, California 91320

SAGE Publications India Pvt Ltd
B 1/I 1 Mohan Cooperative Industrial Area
Mathura Road
New Delhi 110 044

SAGE Publications Asia-Pacific Pte Ltd
33 Pekin Street #02-01
Far East Square
Singapore 048763

Library of Congress Control Number: 2008927532

British Library Cataloguing in Publication data

A catalogue record for this book is available from the British Library

ISBN 978-1-4129-4727-5
ISBN 978-1-4129-4728-2 (pbk)

Typeset by C & M Digitals Pvt Ltd, Chennai, India
Printed and bound in Great Britain by TJ International Ltd, Padstow, Cornwall
Printed on paper from sustainable resources

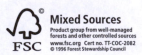

To
Andreas Frangou
Bernard Wallis

Contents

Contributor Profiles

Sid Carter   PhD, MSc, BA, PGCE(A), RNT, RNLD is a Senior School Lecturer in the School of Health and Social Care, Bournemouth University. Sid is a learning disability nurse whose interest in multi-professional working started when teaching both nurses and social workers. This led to an interest in how the cultures of different professions vary so widely, and how this is learnt. Sid's research concerns how emotion can have an impact on learning, using psychophysiological measures.

Rick Fisher   RN, Dip District Nursing Studies PGCE(A) MSc, BA(Hons) is a Senior Lecturer in the School of Social Studies at the University of Chichester. He has many years' experience teaching Community Nursing in Higher Education and has participated as an active member of the Royal College of Nursing Primary Care Educators' Forum, of which he was Chair until 2006. His current research interests as part of his Doctoral Studies are focused around multi-professional relationships and hierarchy in District Nursing practice.

Colin Goble   D.NursSci, MSc, BA Hons, RNLD/DipMH is a Senior Lecturer in Social and Health Care in the School of Social Studies, University of Chichester. Colin's interest in multi-professional working lies mainly in the field of supporting people with learning disabilities to meet their health mental and physical needs – particularly when living in social care settings.

Janet McCray   RN (LD), RNT, BSc, MSc, Phd is a Principal Lecturer in Health and Social Care management, and subject leader for Social and Health Care at the University of Chichester. Janet trained originally as a learning disability nurse, has had a wide range of practice and academic experiences, and has undertaken and published research in the field of inter-and multi-professional learning, leadership and practice.

Ruth Sander   MSc, BA, RN, PGCE is a Senior Lecturer in the School of Health Sciences and Social Work in the Science faculty, University of Portsmouth. Ruth's background is in nursing older people. The interrelated issues that make up the health care needs of older people, make multi-professional working vital. Ruth is Now Senior Lecturer in Health Care Sciences and teaches on courses designed to meet the needs of a wide range of professional groups.

Terry Scragg MA, MPhil, PhD, FCIPD, is a Visiting Fellow in the School of Social Studies, University of Chichester. He has worked in mental health and learning disabilities services in the NHS and social services departments, and has been a non-executive member of two health authorities and a charity trustee both past and present. He is particularly interested in issues of partnership working between the statutory and voluntary sector.

Steve Tee RMN, PGCE, DClinP, BA, MA, Dcp is Associate Director for Post Graduate Education and Senior Lecturer at the School of Nursing and Midwifery, Southampton University. He is also on the executive committee of Solent Mind. He has 20 years' experience of working and publishing in mental health nursing and has held posts in acute, rehabilitation and management positions. His research interests include clinical decision making, user participation and working with people who have long term conditions.

Sandra Wallis PhD, LLM, BA, CQSW is a Senior Lecturer in Social Work at the University of Chichester. Sandra's background is mainly in child protection work, having been a child abuse specialist and child protection conference chair. More recently she has researched social workers' use of evidence in their practice.

Cally Ward MBE BSc (Econ) LSE, MSc Social Work Studies LSE, CQSW is a member of the Valuing People Support Team/CSIP as the national lead for family carers. Prior to that she was the Valuing People Regional Advisor for the West Midlands. Cally was involved in developing one of the first joint degree programmes between nursing and social work at the Southbank University in the 1990s. She was the national coordinator for Positive Futures – looking at ageing and people with learning disabilities and their families.

Acknowledgements

With thanks to all at the University of Chichester for their help, especially Tracy Vine

Introduction

Nursing and Multi-professional Practice is designed to offer nursing students a comprehensive introduction to, and foundation in, multi-professional practice. While the primary market is nursing students, all pre-qualifying professionals will benefit from its central message. The book embraces the swift pace of change and rapid redesign of many services, setting out the new multi-professional partnerships and teams emerging. The intention is to help you understand the reason for the legislative and societal changes that are behind the building of new services and the creation of new contexts of care.

As a student nurse in the twenty-first century, you will be gaining experience in a range of traditional and more innovative practice settings in health and social care. Some of these practice settings will be part of the National Health Service (NHS), for example in acute medicine or in primary care and mental health services, but they may also be in other agencies, like the social care sector, which may provide services to children and families, young people and people with learning disabilities and their families or in the third sector, who currently provide a range of services including foster care, hospice care and drug and alcohol treatment services.

The term third sector describes the range of organisations, independent from government, which occupy the space between the state and the private sector. These include small local community and voluntary groups, registered charities both large and small, foundations, trusts and the growing number of social enterprises and cooperatives (DoH, 2006c). The patients and service users you support may access services from a number of agencies and professionals which you are likely to come into contact with during your placements.

This variety of experiences and breadth of services means that you will be working in a range of teams and require knowledge and understanding of the roles of many different professionals, as well as the types of activity, responsibility and accountability they hold.

This book will introduce you to a number of practice settings in health and social care, describing their purpose and exploring the models of practice that are likely to be in place there. Each chapter will begin with an account of the development of such services describing the societal, technological and economic changes that underpin them. This will be followed by an analysis of the changing nature of the pathway that patients or carers may take when using the service and the likely role of professionals who practise within it.

Central to this exploration will be the multi-professional relationships that take place in the practice setting and the impact on you as a nurse. You will be guided to explore the skills and knowledge you need to work effectively with other professionals and partners to gain the most from the practice experience and achieve successful care for patients, service users and carers.

Throughout the book you will be encouraged to reflect critically on your own knowledge, values, and current and future skill requirements when working with service users and professionals.

The Nursing and Midwifery Council (NMC), the organisation that monitors professional practice of all nurses and midwives, sets out a number of professional skills, knowledge and practice competences required for preparation to practise as a nurse. Programmes that offer pre-registration education for nurses in universities are monitored and measured on the quality of this experience by the Quality Assurance Agency (QAA). A number of statements related to the professional outcomes of such programmes have to be met by all these educational institutions. The intention is that this book will support you in developing subject knowledge related to multi-professional practice outcomes.

Contents

The book is divided into two parts with five chapters in each, Part One is focused on multi-professional practice in predominantly National Health Service settings. Part Two explores broader partnerships beginning with service user and carer perspectives and moving into social care, the third sector and the challenges of leadership in the multi-professional context. Each chapter can be read in sequence or as separate self-contained chapters. The order of content is designed to support your developing practice experiences from the initial focus on what is multi-professional practice culminating in leading teams and the knowledge and skills required to lead and manage others at the end of the book.

Part One

Chapter 1 will introduce the concept of multi-professional practice, offering definitions of multi-professional working, and descriptions of actions involved. Traditional models of multi-professional practice in health and social care and different and more contemporary forms of team working are presented. You will be encouraged to explore the legislative and policy frameworks and the key government agendas and policy drivers behind multi-professional working. **Chapter 2** looks in the same way at nursing, asking you to consider the nature of nursing and what the nurse contributes to the multi-professional care pathway of the patient or service user. **Chapter 3** enables the reader to examine the shift in role of the nurse and likely multi-professional collaborations in primary care. New alliances and challenges for nurses are outlined, providing a foundation to observe further the multi-professional skills of the nurse in the community setting in **Chapter 4**.

Returning to the acute setting, **Chapter 5** highlights the potential new multi-professional and clinical iniatives being established and created by the technological changes in care pathways and for patients with particular health care needs.

Part Two

The key principle here is the focus on multi-professional relationships in a broader context, with a range of external stakeholders, and where the nurse is a significant linchpin of the partnership work taking place. **Chapter 6** looks at the needs of the service user and carer within new service design models located in services for people with learning difficulty. The challenge of meeting an individual's complex needs and ensuring rights and wishes are met are central to the discussion. Often when care is provided individuals' needs and wishes may be compromised and professional and multi-professional intervention contested. Two areas of practice where this is also significant are mental health care, highlighted in **Chapter 7**, and children's services, which are examined in **Chapter 8**. In these settings the intervention of professionals and multi-professional collaboration may be viewed with ambivalence, created through the necessary but often unwanted concern in terms of child protection, and the legal aspects of care for people with severe mental illness. Once again legislation and ideological views on what is viewed as an appropriate service drive multi-professional practice and hence the discussion and analysis here. **Chapter 9** takes into account the growing third sector. The sector is described and likely roles and alliances are offered as examples of new types of partnerships. Finally, recognising the increasingly complex nature of all these new roles and associations, **Chapter 10** sets out the leadership strategies needed for good practice and effective multi-professional activity.

Helping you learn

Throughout the book you will find a range of helpful learning activities to develop your knowledge further. You will find:

- Guided study activity linked to the practice context being explored with pointers to help you.

    The purpose of this is twofold. First, to provide a review of your reading and understanding of the content to that point in the text and, second, to encourage you to bring and apply the new theory being presented to your practice experience.

- Practice setting case studies or examples to give a context for the theory presented.

These case studies will offer you a further example of multi-professional working as an additional aid, and will help you if you have not worked in the particular setting being described.

- The book also includes:
  - Websites to link content and topics presented in each chapter.
  - A full bibliography of evidenced material.

  These will help you to evidence your assessed work in formal assignments.

I hope you enjoy this book and it enables you to think in more depth about working in partnership with other professionals and service users and carers.

Janet McCray

PART I

1

Preparing for Multi-professional Practice
Janet McCray

By reading this chapter you should be able to:

- **define what is meant by multi-professional practice**
- **identify the drivers towards multi-professional practice**
- **describe how people work together**
- **identify present barriers to multi-professional working and how they may be overcome**
- **reflect on your experience of multi-professional working at this stage in your practice**
- **access websites to learn more about models of multi-professional working and new professional roles.**

Introduction

Working with other professionals is part of everyday practice in health and social care. Multi-professional collaboration and team work have been presented as positive and necessary practice interventions, to achieve good care provision by successive governments for several decades.

This endorsement can be viewed in a number of ways. At one level, politicians have been responding to outcomes of major inquiries into child abuse, where all too often relationships and communication strategy between professionals and agencies have been criticised (Laming, 2003). From a different perspective responses are focused around a need to provide a more holistic and person-centred approach to care provision from service providers. Founded in the move from institutional models of care to community based services that has taken place is a desire to cut down the need for service users and their families to be constantly assessed and in contact with a huge number of different professionals. It takes into account both the need for a person-centred approach to practice and the need to maximise the use of resources in service delivery.

While it would be difficult to argue with these aims, and successive governments and national bodies have attempted to achieve them, there is evidence that working with other professionals has not always been straightforward or effective. This does not mean good multi-professional practice does not take place, rather that it can be a more complex process than we might expect.

In order to help you make sense of the challenges faced, this chapter will begin by examining what is meant by multi-professional practice. Traditional and more radical models of multi-professional practice will be defined; while key characteristics of it – such as team working and team work activity – will be reviewed. The perspectives of researchers and professionals from a range of health and social care disciplines will be presented. As part of this process the chapter will explore why people work together, and offer examples of the legislative frameworks and policy drivers that have influenced developments. Having established *why* people work together, you will be guided to consider *how* people work together, and the forms of teamwork roles they may use. The chapter study activity will support you through the content presented here and, throughout, you will be encouraged to reflect on what is needed to make multi-professional practice work.

Towards a definition of multi-professional practice

A number of terms have been used to describe professionals working together. You may be familiar with the following: multi-professional, multi-disciplinary, multi-agency, inter-professional, inter-agency, collaboration and partnership working. Leathard (1994: 5) describes the 'terminological quagmire' created as developments in practice have accelerated. In her analysis of terms, Leathard (1994: 6) suggests that for some professionals the use of inter-professional is not adequate as it applies to only two professional groups working together, whereas multi-professional infers a wider group. Pollard et al. (2005: 10 cited in McCray, 2007a) define multi-professional practice as practice between different professional groups but not necessarily including collaboration. This means that professional groups may agree with a family or patient on an intervention, but each professional group will work separately to provide the care agreed. Carrier and Kendall (1995: 10) suggest that inter-professional work may be more conducive to working across boundaries to meet client needs.

You may have noted in health care practice settings the use of the term multi-disciplinary team, used as an alternative term to multi- or inter-professional practice. Leathard notes (1994: 6) that it is usually used to describe a team of individuals from different professional backgrounds 'who share common objectives but who make a different but complementary contribution to practice' (Leathard, 1994: 6). Sheehan, et al. (2007: 18) cite Paul and Peterson (2001) and offer three distinctive teamwork approaches in health care. These are multi-disciplinary, where interaction and communication across teams tends to be informal as in Leathard's (1994: 6) definition; interdisciplinary, where the roles of professionals overlap and communication is formal and informal for the good of the patient; and transdisciplinary, where there is greater overlap, blending and blurring of professional roles. Transdisciplinary team work is the least common approach currently in place in the NHS in the UK.

In social care settings, for example in family social work teams, the term multi-agency may be used. This term describes multi-professional practice in teams with the involvement of a range of services such as education, housing and health, and professionals including social workers, nurses, teachers and housing workers, all involved in providing services for an individual (McCray, 2007b). Increasingly, the service user and carer and their representative will also be a part of this multi-agency work and this may be called partnership working. Changes in how services are delivered set out in policy documents by government are often the key driver for these types of activity, although good informal practice may also be in place. Three models of multi-agency working are offered in the *Every Child Matters* guidance (DFES, 2006).

First, a multi-agency panel in which:

- Practitioners remain employed by their home agency.
- They meet as a panel or network on a regular basis to discuss children with additional needs who would benefit from multi-agency input.
- In some panels, case work is carried out by panel members. Other panels take a more strategic role, employing key workers to lead on case work. This might be viewed as multi-professional working.

Second, a multi-agency team where:

- There is a more formal configuration than a panel, with practitioners seconded or recruited into the team.
- The team has a leader and works to a common purpose and common goals.
- Practitioners may maintain links with their home agencies through supervision and training.

These are in place in Youth Offending teams in children's services and are an example of inter-professional working.

Finally, an integrated service which would include:

- A range of separate services that share a common location, and work together in a collaborative way.
- A visible service hub for the community.
- A management structure that facilitates integrated working.

This type of working is the most radical in terms of working across professional boundaries and is closer to the transdisciplinary team working model described above, with an emphasis on formal collaboration.

Collaboration in the form of partnership working across organisations or agencies in health or social care may be an element of multi-professional and multi-agency activity. This consists of a formal arrangement within which collaboration and collaborative practice are agreed through contractual agreements. Other less formal models may be in place. Collaborative working can be defined as:

> A respect for other professionals and service users and their skills and from this starting point, an agreed sharing of authority, responsibility and resources for specific outcomes or actions, gained through cooperation and consensus. (McCray, 2007a: 132)

So let us now return to our starting aim, which was to define multi-professional working. Your reading so far has shown that there are a number of terms used in practice by professionals to describe multi-professional working often to mean the same thing. You have read that a number of academics have explored the reasons for this. To help you use this book effectively, the term multi-professional will be used by all chapter writers, because:

- it is used most predominantly and commonly in the literature and by professionals in practice across the NHS and broader practice contexts in the same way.
- the most important elements of multi-professional practice activity are collaboration and teamwork, which are at the centre of service provision and good care and which will be the key focus of your reading and activity throughout this book.

Now let's consider the design of service delivery models in place in practice settings. There are varying degrees of multi-professional collaboration taking place depending on the sort of care and support being delivered to whom, and the types of team in place. Reviewing the impetus and purpose behind these models of service delivery will enable you to understand further the nature of multi-professional working and help you answer the question 'Why do people work together?'

Why people work together: drivers for multi-professional practice

Ultimately, changes in the way funding of services is allocated by government in order to make their policies happen, means services must develop new ways of working with other professionals to continue to maintain funding. This is a significant factor in the shift towards multi-professional working. There are a number of reasons for this, which are discussed below.

Protecting vulnerable people

The need to ensure a more effective safety net for protection of vulnerable people in society in the light of public responses to child abuse cases. For example, the need for policy makers to address the recommendations of public inquiries where key failures had occurred around professional accountability and communication, as in the case of Victoria Climbié (Laming, 2003). This has led to a radical review and a radical transformation of professional practice in children's services. Every Child Matters (DFES, 2004) made recommendations about children's services which were formally built on the Children Act (DFES, 2004), setting out five core outcomes for children. These outcomes are charged to the local authority who must meet the requirements of section 10 of the Children Act, to secure collaboration 'through the creation of a single children's and young people plan (CYPP), leading to the creation of children's trust' (DFES, 2005). The breadth of these outcomes means a multi-agency approach is needed, and multi-professional practice will be at the centre of ensuring changes are made to services so that these outcomes can be met and funding streams follow.

Changes to models of service delivery based on ideological issues

These can be seen in the move from institutional to community-based services for service users with mental health or learning disabilities, culminating in a need for different working relationships among professionals and with service users and carers. In mental health services, community provision has meant that some individuals with severe mental illness living in the community may be at increased risk of physical health problems, as they are reliant on attending primary care services which may not always be most accessible for this group of people. The document *Choosing Health: Supporting the Physical Needs of People with Severe Mental Illness – Commissioning Framework* (DoH, 2006d), sets out the core issues involved in improving provision and subsequently care. Advocating a nurse-led assessment service are a number of multi-agency and multi-professional relationships required to improve services. The introduction and further development of individual budgets for service users in social care will increase the collaborative and partnership element of multi-professional practice as the service user drives the delivery and design of his or her needs.

Transformation of acute health care delivery created by technological change

The massive technological changes in operating practice in acute medicine such as keyhole surgery, and evidence-based management of post-operative conditions has made the patient journey through secondary health care a much shorter one. Patients can be discharged rapidly following intervention that can aid recovery time and ensure maximum bed occupation in acute care wards. Such changing practice means the patient and his or her family has a greater reliance on the primary care team post operatively. Multi-professional relationships between secondary and primary care health services are crucial, as are those within the primary care health team, post discharge.

Transition of management of people with long term chronic conditions to the community

A move towards community-based support for patients with long term chronic conditions has taken place with support provided though community-based nursing teams in liaison with GP practices. The management of these processes from referral to assessment through to ongoing management is usually led by community nursing teams with a centrally led administrative function. A number of multi-professional networks are needed for this service to work effectively involving primary and secondary health care services, social care agencies and the independent sector.

The changing role of the voluntary and independent sectors

As care of elderly people has moved to the community, local authorities are increasingly working in formal partnerships with a third sector service that will be commissioned to deliver social care support to older people living at home or in residential care. Additionally, primary care trusts in health care may work in partnership with a third sector hospice, commissioning them to provide day-care for people requiring palliative care. Frequently, service users groups and their representatives are integral members of these formal partnerships and teams involved in the planning and design of packages of care. Professionals working in teams within these partnership agreements have both a formal and informal working relationship on which to deliver multi-professional practice. Commissioning arrangements may be very challenging, due to expectations of high quality delivery of service despite tight resources.

Guided Study 1.1

Think about a recent day in practice and the experience of a patient or service user you met.

Ask yourself:

- Is this patient's experience likely to have changed in recent times?
- What would have created this change?
- Do these changes bring about different roles for professionals?
- Has the role of the nurse changed?
- What multi-professional roles and relationships might be created?

The section above should help you to answer the question in Guided Study 1.1 and, from your reading here and practice experience, you will have seen that service delivery models are influenced by a number of factors. Multi-professional practice can occur in a number of ways and to a number of levels. Traditional and emerging ways of working may be in place involving professionals in health care, health and social care, and increasingly education, health and social care. The pace of change is unprecedented. Narrow definitions of primary care and of team working can no longer be regarded as the norm as complex care and intervention takes place within community settings, and social care is undergoing radical transformation.

In forthcoming chapters you will read and consider case study-based examples of these changes in practice. First we continue to discuss these newly developing models of service in order to answer the question 'How do people work together?'

How people work together

Most multi-professional work takes place in a team work setting. Mickan and Roger (2000: 201) define a team as a small number of members with appropriate skills to complete a specific task, with agreed performance goals and collective responsibility for achieving them. However, there are many levels and types of multi-professional team working and collaboration with increasingly innovative models of practice.

Much of the research into multi-professional practice has taken place in health care Odegard (2007: 46) cites Barr, et al. (2005) and Doherty (1995) who observes that multi-professional collaboration may involve several health care levels, including with organisations, service users, carers and communities as well as professionals. Doherty (1995) explores the scale of collaboration among professionals in health care, from level 1 minimum – professionals based in separate places and separate case loads through to level 5 – where all professionals are fully integrated, share offices, cases and totally understand each other's professional roles and values. At level 5 the team and its functioning is important, as are patient issues. In Doherty's research most professionals were collaborating at level 3, sharing the same systems and meeting face to face to discuss patients and their care. However, new models of practice – such as integrated teams in adult care services – mean that level 5 collaboration is becoming more frequent. An evaluation by Hudson (2007: 8) of the Sedgefield integrated team, from 2004 to mid-2006, describes the development of five locality based teams. These new teams incorporated three partners, the primary health care trust, borough councils for housing and the county council for social care services. Service models were created which were both locally based and with integrated teams at level 5 in terms of collaboration. Hudson, in his analysis of the Sedgefield evaluation findings (2007: 4), presents two models of teamwork based on a review of the literature, each holding two distinct sets of characteristics. These models are identified as the *pessimistic* and *optimistic* models. The pessimistic model (Hudson, 2007: 4) includes a distinctiveness of trait, knowledge, power, accountability and culture, in contrast to the optimistic model, where team members share a commonality of values, accountability, learning, location, culture and case.

In reviewing these two models, the terms *traditional* and *contemporary* might also be appropriate to describe the different positions of professions within teams. Traditional team working in the pessimistic model may be straitjacketed by barriers that professionals holding distinctive trait, knowledge, status, power, accountability and culture created. Yet contemporary or optimistic model characteristics suggest that, as Hudson notes, 'features that professions have in common may outweigh factors that divide them' (Hudson, 2007: 5).

In answering the question: 'How do people work together?', it is worth exploring Hudson's research more fully. First, in relation to values, McCray (2007b: 254) describes personal values as 'something that individuals hold at the centre of their being. Values are developed over time and from experience, and personal values may reflect an individual's culture, moral stance or lifestyle.' Hudson (2007: 5) suggests that team working offers the opportunity to share values based on a belief in universalism; that is, services for all and benevolence in service delivery. In terms of influencing how people work together, values may be very significant, as shared beliefs might be a huge motivator for collaboration, overcoming the differences created by professional traits, knowledge, status and power for the good of the patient or service user. Such differences may be created by the set of behaviors, authority, separate and specialised knowledge (Hudson, 2007: 5) that have been developed historically by some professions and which may contribute to a monopoly of views and practice specialisms that ensure maintenance of the profession as paramount.

Second, in relation to the commonality of case, Hudson citing Guy (1986) writes that as patient or service user need becomes more complex, there is a greater urgency to involve a range of professionals, which we discussed earlier in relation to changes to children's services. Such changes mean that joint responsibility for cases means there is less room for individual professional contribution and more support for multi-professional collaboration.

Hudson also notes in his review that a shared location may also be a key factor in how people work together as team members. Thus leading to socialisation to a team, rather than to a separate profession.

Summarising, Hudson (2007: 14) notes that there is much to be gained from the optimistic model, particularly among some professional groups. Key factors identified in his study and highlighted here can assist in the further development and integration of teams and impact on service user outcomes and safety. They can also help us to address the question of how professionals work together as we continue to explore professional roles in teams.

Guided Study 1.2

From your reading so far, what factors may make a difference to how people work together?

You could have included:

- Shared values and shared beliefs about service delivery
- Shared responsibility and accountability for care
- Meeting face to face to discuss cases
- Shared environment.

Roles in teams

By exploring team roles, we can look at research from two positions; the team leadership role and the team player role. Let's start with leadership.

Leadership

Our opening study, by Hean et al. (2006: 161), involves health and social care students entering university. Ten professional groups rated each other on a number of characteristics which could have an impact on future team roles. One of the main purposes of the research was to investigate the impact of previously held stereotypes on perceptions of professional group characteristics. The findings are of interest when we start to think about team roles in practice. For example midwives, nurses and social workers were rated highest on interpersonal characteristics and doctors and pharmacists lowest, which was also the case when being a team player was rated.

When leadership was scored doctors were most highly rated with midwives and social workers also viewed highly. Hean et al. (2006: 177) note an assumption that is made that fits with other studies and with their own perception identified by Freeman et al. (2000) below, that doctors are natural leaders.

The authors of this research with undergraduate professionals write that it will be interesting to note if these views remain after the students have participated in a shared multi-professional education experience or into practice on qualification. Equally, such views are debated in terms of the challenge facing some professional groups – such as nurses – who are required and are often best placed to take on leadership roles in team settings.

Moving onward to qualified professionals, Sheehan et al. (2007: 18) cite Freeman et al. (2000), who define a number of teamwork philosophies or characteristics held by teamwork members in health care. These individual perspectives show the range of different views of teamwork roles held by professionals. In their study, doctors saw themselves as having a directive role: seeing themselves as leaders of teams. Social workers, nurses and therapists viewed their role as collaborators and team players and Freeman et al. described this role as integrative (2000). A further perspective was that of the elective team member: someone who was largely autonomous with limited contact with other team members, for instance mental health workers.

It would seem that roles established early are maintained into practice in health care in a number of teamwork settings. What's more, in acute clinical practice, many traditional teams of clinicians are hierarchial. Bleakley et al. (2006: 468) studied team roles in operating theatres, where they observed that technical expertise determined leadership and decision making processes, even though when mistakes were made it was usually due to communication or other non-technical skills.

Sheehan et al. (2007: 19) caution against always assuming that doctors dominate team decisions and take on the leadership role. They cite Unsworth et al.'s (1997) study in a rehabilitation setting, where occupational therapists were as significant in decision making as doctors. Moreover Gair and Hartery (2001, cited by Sheehan et al., 2007: 19) write that doctors were more likely to have their proposals questioned than any other professional group and were willing to concede and accept alternative decisions. Recent changes to qualifying education (DoH, 2004c) means that doctors will be focusing on their leadership and management development as well as clinical skills from foundation placement after medical school (www.mmc.nhs.uk/pages/specialities/specialityframework), which may change the way in which they negotiate and work with others in teams.

In health care services we can see some interesting research findings and educational responses to multi-professional roles, notably about perception in terms of who should lead teams and what the basis for these views is. Hean et al. (2006: 178), when discussing their findings, see early perceptions of professional roles as both potentially harmonious and a source of conflict in teamwork, if expectations of other professionals are not met. A range of other factors can also influence leadership roles, such as organisational structures which might make team working very formal, and the type and duration of the teamwork activity underway. For example, if you have worked in an acute hospital ward you will know that some practice processes – such as the assessment of older people – may be very complex and linked to a set of procedures which work on a step to step basis. As steps are in effect 'ticked off' and the patient is moved through the system there is little room for multi-professional contributions (Huby et al., 2007), which could be viewed as a result of a hierchial medical leadership model. In reality it's the process of assessment itself that creates the lack of participation.

In work across health and social care it is possible that change may be more challenging if ideas about professional roles are very deeply held, especially when it comes to team leadership. New models of young people's services mean that some managers in social care are now leading health care professionals in drug crisis teams. This should bring extra opportunities for face-to-face multi-professional communication and information sharing to enhance good practice, yet a common concern of social care managers is the medical model of practice these professionals will bring to the team. If we return to Hean et al.'s research (2006: 161), the origin of views about professional practice of health care professionals came from very early professional experiences. Assumptions made about professional roles and the dangers of seeing uniform values within any one professional group and professional culture may create unnecessary barriers and inhibit multi-professional collaboration and change.

Guided Study 1.3

Return to a recent practice experience and a patient or service user you met.

- Where were they receiving care or support and which professionals were giving it?
- What agency did the professionals work for?
- How many professionals seemed to be involved?
- Who was leading the care and support and why do you think this was the case?
- What agency was funding the care and support?
- What role did the nurse have?

Need to know more?

In completing the activity where you able to answer all sections? Do you need more information about practice? If so make a note of areas you need to explore further, on your next day in practice.

Being a team player

Earlier in the chapter, Freeman et al. described the collaborative role in multi-professional practice as integrative (2000), meaning having a purposeful role in how the team works. This role is often the domain of nurses and therapists in health care. A team player role is significant because those professionals who take it on have a commitment to the team function and its processes. This means their focus on communicating with their team members as part of meeting team objectives and providing feedback after and during intervention keeps the team together and ensures the meeting of client or service user need.

Research shows us that other professionals also invest in the team player role. In children's services, Odegard's Norwegian study (2007: 52) measured time spent on collaboration by professionals in a child mental health team. The researchers asked nine professional groups including teachers, nurses, social workers and psychologists, to measure how much time they spent on collaboration within their own organisation and outside it, in a working day. Odegard found that all professionals studied stated they spent on average 40 per cent of their time collaborating with others in their own organisation about the children's needs, while social workers spent the most time collaborating both internally and externally.

Mickan and Rodgers' study (2005: 358) explored the characteristics of effective teams in health care. The importance of team cohesion was noted by participants in the study and the camaraderie and involvement that was generated in team working created commitment to the team and other members (2005: 366), resulting in a number of positive aspects for practice.

Some roles in practice formally merge leadership and team player roles, as teams and networks cross from secondary care to primary care and health and social care in the community. An example of this is the community matron. Community matrons work in multi-professional, multi-agency settings. They therefore need a high level of communication, problem-solving and decision-making skills as well as advanced clinical skills. They must be able to manage risk appropriately, and to take responsibility for leading complex care coordination, professional practice and leadership, underpinned by multi-agency and partnership working. In social care, a children's centre manager – for example in a Sure Start project – will also combine leadership and team player roles working with local communities to determine priorities for children from an early age, as well as working with other professionals and partners to meet strategic performance objectives in relation to the educational, social and health care needs of children.

Guided Study 1.4

The role of the community matron and a children's centre manager are set out above. What sort of service users, carers and professionals might they work with? What multi-professional knowledge and skills will they require to undertake this role?

(Continued)

Need to know more?

In completing the activity, were you able to answer all of the questions? Do you need more information about these roles in practice? If you do, make a note of the areas you need to explore further on your next day in practice.

The following websites will help you:

For Children's Centre Managers: www.surestart.gov.uk/research/
For Community Matrons: www.dh.gov.uk/en/Publicationsandstatistics/Publications/
    PublicationsPolicyAndGuidance/DH_4133997
www.nmc-uk.org.uk website encourages joint working in children's services

The roles of community matron and children's centre manager merge multi-professional leadership and team player skills and knowledge. Yet their roles could not be effective if the views of service users and communities were not seen as essential in decision making and planning about service delivery and forms of practice intervention.

Service user involvement

Attempting to describe one model of meaningful service user involvement in multi-professional practice is just not possible. Beresford (2005: 8) cites his earlier work with Croft (Beresford and Croft, 1996) to offer the two most widely used interpretations. First, the managerialist approach, which focuses on getting service users to inform service design and provision. Second is the democratic approach, which may be service user-led and attempts to give more control to service users over the services they use and how they use them. The democratic approach is more concerned with gaining power for service users, while the managerialist approach is more about information gathering.

In terms of multi-professional practice and collaboration, it is likely that service users will be involved in both managerialist and democratic roles in teamwork. Service user groups will be consulted or co-opted to teams to plan and evaluate service changes in primary care, fulfilling a largely managerialist agenda. Equally, a multi-professional team may seek the individual view of a young person who is a service user on the type of foster care he or she would like, which should be a more democratic model of participation.

As a nurse you will be aware that people's state of physical and emotional health could impact on their level of participation in decision making about their care. Likewise in social care, in child protection cases some families are unlikely to willingly participate in decisions that may involve taking their children into care. Other service users may not seem able to communicate their wishes, for example people with learning disability or older people who have cognitive impairment.

This does not mean that the individual's views need not be explored in team decision making, but that you should be aware of how some systems in health and social care prevent participation from being as effective as it could be. If you revisit Huby et al.'s (2007: 64) research about discharge planning in older peoples services, you will see that they note that the very specific criteria used to tick off stages in discharge which prevented multi-professional collaboration also inhibited patient participation. They note that simple changes to the planning process could make a difference.

In multi-professional working, good practice should include a discussion about the nature of the role of the service user in the team decision-making process. Does the team see the contribution of individual service users to activity as holding more, less or equal value than professional input? Are there difficulties in involving the service user patient or carer and how could these be overcome? Is the team making assumptions about what people might choose? From an open debate real collaboration and practice to create change or challenge current systems can take place.

Developing your knowledge, skills and values

You can see from the research that multi-professional working takes place because of several drivers. People work together in teams in differing roles to meet key objectives. A number of positive characteristics for teams have been identified. As you have read the chapter content and worked through the guided study exercises you will be gaining or building on your knowledge of multi-professional working. You have identified key skills, knowledge and values to make multi-professional practice work.

Guided Study 1.5

Make a note of the positive characteristics, key skills and knowledge required for multi-professional practice below.

You could have included:

- Sharing values and beliefs about service delivery
- Sharing responsibility and accountability for care
- Meeting face to face to discuss cases
- Sharing a working environment
- Working with a team to engage service users in a meaningful way
- Avoiding common perceptions of other professional groups and their role in teams
- Making collaboration a major part of your working day
- Building strong team relationships and strong links with the community and or other services
- Communicating with team members about meeting team goals
- Learning about other professional roles
- Being aware of some practice processes such as discharge planning that may inhibit multi-professional team working and patient or service user involvement
- Leadership skills.

Conclusion

This chapter has introduced you to the concept of multi-professional practice, where the motivators for its use have come from, and how and why people work together.

By concentrating on what is needed for good practice you have been guided to identify some barriers to multi-professional working, which can make practice ineffective. You will know that by not addressing gaps in your knowledge, skills and values and any strongly held misconceptions of other professionals, service users and their roles, you may not be as well equipped as you could be for twenty-first century practice. The forthcoming chapters will explore these themes further, linking to specific aspects and models of service delivery and helping you to increase your knowledge and identify skills to use to develop your practice.

2

Nursing and Multi-professional Practice
Ruth Sander

By reading this chapter you should be able to:

- **define the professional discipline of nursing**
- **describe the role of the nurse in supporting patients, service users and carers**
- **recognise what makes nursing distinctive in the multi-professional team setting**
- **move towards a further understanding of the tensions nurses face in the multi-professional health care setting**
- **reflect on the type and focus of multi-professional action in nursing practice through a case study example**
- **access website links to learn more about the profession of nursing.**

Introduction

Cooperation with others within the team is one of the central pillars of the Nursing and Midwifery Council's Code of Professional Practice (NMC, 2004). The code makes clear that nurses must not only respect the skills, expertise and contribution of their colleagues but also give those colleagues the benefit of their own knowledge, skill and expertise for the benefit of their patients. This is a two-way process; the patient's interests are best served by a nurse who values the role of other health care providers but is also confident about his or her own skills and prepared to make his or her voice heard in order to make a full contribution within the team.

Quality Assurance Agency Benchmark statements, which describe the nature and characteristics of study and training for student nurses, include the statement that the award holder should 'contribute with skill and confidence to effective multi-professional/multi-agency working' (QAA, 2001: 16). Nurses cannot work in isolation. The health care arena is increasingly complex so cooperation with other specialists is vital.

Nurses work in many different and very diverse settings; they work in schools, in industry, in hospitals and the community; they work on advice lines, private clinics and care homes. In each setting they will be working with a different professional team and have a different function within the team. The purpose of this chapter is to outline some of the different roles nurses take and look at the different positions and relationships within the team that may result.

This chapter will help you to examine the contribution that nurses can make to the multi-professional team. You will be encouraged to explore the different roles that the nurse can play within the team and, through a case study, how their place within the team changes as the needs of the patient change.

Defining nursing

To fully explore the place of the nurse in the multi-professional team you must first understand the role of the nurse. This is harder than it seems. The government is currently reviewing the role of the nurse and nurse education to meet the changing requirements of society and service in the NHS. They intend to 'build a consensus about the role of the nurse, find meaningful ways to improve the quality of nursing care and identify those accountable for improving it, modernise nursing education and career pathways and recruiting and retaining the best candidates to nursing' (DoH, 2008a: 18). All of this activity is very new, but one thing we can be sure of is that the nurse is central to health care, whatever the situation. The nurse is always responsible for promoting comfort, both physical and emotional, but that is never the limit of the role. It may also include:

- *Education for a healthy lifestyle.* This may mean encouraging children to take appropriate exercise and eat a well balanced diet; it may mean helping young people to avoid the dangers of drugs and to understand safe sex; it may be helping people to give up smoking or alcohol abuse or it may be helping children or adults to cope with the long term effects of disease such as diabetes or heart failure. As well as his or her background knowledge, the nurse must understand the role of the dietician, pharmacist, doctor, social worker or any other professional and the part they play in maintaining health.
- *Coordinating care.* The nurse remains central to the person's health experience while other professionals tend to move in and out as circumstances change. Dieticians, occupational therapists, physiotherapists, medical technicians, speech therapists and many other professional groups will become central for a while and, when their task is completed, will again become peripheral. The nurse is very often the professional who remains throughout the patient's journey and so is ideally placed to coordinate the input of the others.
- *Supporting therapy.* Sometimes the way that the nurse can best help his or her patient is by continuing regimes prescribed by other members of the multi-professional team. This may, for instance, mean ensuring that a programme established by a physiotherapist is

continued throughout the day or that medication is administered as prescribed by a doctor.

- *Giving technical care.* The nurse is also a skilled technician, understanding and operating the complex equipment that may be part of the patient experience. In some specialities nurses will be performing highly complex invasive procedures as the central figure in a supportive multi-professional team; or at other times the nurse may use technical equipment to supply diagnostic information for other team members to use.
- *Diagnosis and treatment.* In some circumstances nurses will be responsible for diagnosing health related problems, requesting investigations or input from other members of the inter-professional team and overseeing treatment given.
- *Care giving.* Care is a notoriously difficult concept to define. McCance (2005) suggests that it involves 'serious attention' and 'providing for'. In this role nurses provide the link between the patient and whichever other professional is best able to support their needs at that moment.

With such a broad range of roles the nurse could be forgiven for struggling for a clear sense of identity. There have been many attempts to define nursing but perhaps the best known remains that of Virginia Henderson:

> The unique function of the nurse is to assist the individual, sick or well, in the performance of those activities contributing to health or its recovery (or to a peaceful death) that he would perform unaided if he had the necessary strength, will or knowledge. And to do this in such a way as to help him gain independence as rapidly as possible. (1966: 8)

The quality assurance agency (QAA, 2001: 6) recognises the need to define nursing in order to develop benchmarks for education. They describe nursing as a discipline that:

> Focuses on promoting health and helping individuals, families and groups to meet their health needs. Nursing work involves assisting people whose autonomy is impaired, who may present with a range of disabilities or health related problems; to perform a range of activities, sometimes acting for, or on behalf of the patient. A defining feature of nursing is that it provides twenty-four hour care with a focus on meeting people's intimate needs

The important thing about these definitions is that they say, in effect, that the nurse will do what is needed when it is needed. There are no clear boundaries to the role and nor should there be. The nurse works with the professional who is most appropriate to the patient at that time in the way that is most appropriate in that situation. This may mean making detailed assessments to provide autonomous care or it may mean incorporating plans designed by others. The only thing that is important is that the needs of the patient remain central to the nurse's decisions.

So what is the role of the nurse in relation to other health and social care professionals? There are large areas of overlap but the nurse and the tasks the nurse might perform, both autonomously and in the support of others, are too numerous and develop and alter too rapidly for them to be listed. But at the core of the question 'What is nursing?' is the concern to help the individual, in whichever way is made appropriate by the situation, to achieve health or comfort.

The nurse as care giver

A defining feature of nursing is that it provides care with a focus on meeting people's intimate needs (QAA, 2001). No nurse should ever shy away from the caring role – sometimes called basic nursing care. Bjorkstrom et al. (2006) found that student nurses asked to describe their role gave 'to care for others' as the most frequent response and that this view was consistent throughout their training. Henderson (2006) tries to identify what are the key features of nursing by examining the way in which the lay person would see the nurse. Sifting through various definitions, she comes to the conclusion that the only universally held idea of nursing is that it 'embodies the characteristic of a service that is intimate, constant and comforting'. The importance of this work in supporting the activities of other health professionals should never be underestimated. The skills of the nurse in providing health and nourishment are vital if the plans of the multi-professional team are to be effective. Henderson (2006) reflects on the words of Florence Nightingale, who is often said to have founded professional nursing. She believed that, in the end, only nature could cure; doctors can remove some of the obstructions with their medicine or surgery but that is all they can do. Once they have done that they rely on nature and it is the nurse who can do most to support nature by putting the patient in the 'best condition for nature to act upon him'. The good nurse will ensure the required cleanliness, nutrition, elimination and comfort that puts the body in the best position to heal itself. Without these vital, but often little acclaimed, skills the efforts of other professionals would often be in vain. Performing intimate care while maintaining dignity and communicating effectively regardless of physiological or emotional barriers requires every bit as much knowledge and skill as performing the most technical of tasks and is equally important if health is to be regained. Richman et al. (2005) found that higher levels of hope were associated with a decreased likelihood of having or developing a disease. The nurse needs to be happy to take whichever role is in the best interest of his or her patient at that particular moment.

The 24-hour role of the nurse

Henderson (2006) emphasised the importance of the 24-hour availability of the nurse and sees the fact that it is 'constant' as one of its central characteristics. The QAA (2001) also list one of the defining features of nursing as the fact that it provides 24-hour care. This is a core feature of the nurse's role in relationship to the multi-professional team because, if the nurse alone is available, then he or she must be able to cover for the role of any other health provider. Kitson believes that it is this 24-hour commitment that 'sets nursing apart from other health care professionals and links it more closely to the type of surveillance and care given to an ill or dependent person at home' (Kitson, 2003).

While Henderson (2006) believed that providing intimate care is what unites nurses from all specialities, she also states that nurses may have to 'supply other types of service when the physician, the physical therapist, the social worker or other health provider is unavailable'. This puts nurses in a pivotal position. It is not a reciprocal relationship: other professionals do not always need to understand the intricacies of the nurse's role as the nurse is always available but if the nurse does not understand the role of other therapists then their plans cannot be woven into the 24-hour routine. The occupational therapist on a rehabilitation ward, for instance, may prescribe adapted cutlery but it is the nurse who will be available at each mealtime to ensure that it is correctly used.

Other professionals expect nurses to step into their shoes when they cannot attend but do not expect to turn a hand to that intimate and personal care that is seen as the unifying function of the nurse. While support workers (who work under various titles such as care assistant, nursing assistant) will share the intimate and personal care giving and many routine technical tasks, they are not expected to have the overview of health needs that allows the nurse to cover for absent members of the multi-professional team.

The nurse as autonomous practitioner

Autonomy plays an important part in nurses' job satisfaction but the literature shows that they are often dissatisfied with this aspect of their work and want greater autonomy in decision making (Mrayyan, 2004). Autonomy is affected by several factors, one of which is the relationship with doctors. Nursing has traditionally been seen as being partially dependent on medicine. McCray (2007b) describes nurses as 'semi-autonomous practitioners' working to guidelines drawn up by doctors. This is often a necessary and highly effective element of multi-professional working. However, nurses are independent professionals and there may be times when a doctor-led scenario is not in the patient's best interest, but remains in place through issues of power and status. This can be problematic because, as McCray points out, doctors may have difficulty taking advice from other health care professionals, whereas nurses may lack the confidence to challenge their authority. Manias and Street (2001) found that doctors use nurses to supplement their information during ward rounds but are reluctant to allow them to participate in decision making.

Relationships between doctors and nurses have never been simple. Status, pay, education and gender have a strong influence on the relationship. Historically, doctors have been expected to be autonomous and independent while nursing traditions have encouraged rule-following. Despite these differences the nurse–doctor relationship is at the centre of health care delivery (Jones, 2003) so it is vital that the relationship is developed in the way that best suits the patient's needs. While harmony is extremely important, where the nurse is more experienced and knowledgeable or better placed to understand a particular patient's needs and wishes, then accepting a subservient role is in nobody's best interest.

There is a pattern of behaviour between nurses and doctors that has been described as the doctor–nurse game (Jones, 2003). The nature of the relationship between these two professional groups has led nurses to be reluctant to overtly make a diagnosis even when their greater experience has meant that they are better placed to do this than the doctor they are working with. Instead they will offer advice or provide information in such a way that both parties can act as if the diagnosis was made by the doctor. This ensures that the authority of the doctor is not challenged and avoids open conflict but can lead to poor communication and perpetuates a view that nurses are unable to lead in clinical situations.

To be fully effective in multi-professional teams and give patients the full advantage of their skills, nurses need to resist these stereotypical behaviour patterns. Experienced nurses have expertise that can be important in the decision-making process and this is being recognised in clinical situations such as in decision making around resuscitation (Baskett et al., 2005). Gradually, the nursing profession is developing new educational and organisational structures that challenge what Diaski (2004) describes as 'disempowering discourses and practices' among nurses. Equally, the new Modernising Medical Careers Curriculum for Doctors will emphasise the need for doctors to work more actively to negotiate roles in team work settings (NHS, 2006).

The nurse as team member and team leader

To truly provide support, the nurse must be aware of the functioning of the organisation as a whole and the potential struggles within it. Only with an understanding of the whole picture can the nurse hope to support the patient. The whole concept of support becomes the product of interaction and relationships with the multi-professional team rather than a simple relationship between nurse and patient.

Ellis et al. (2005: 276), when examining the concept of nursing support, discuss the complexity of providing this in a health care system where they must interact with massive numbers of people. The nurse does not operate independently but only as part of a health care system that is very complex. They point out that the many professionals involved in the system will have varying objectives and that the search for power may play a part in relationships. To truly provide support the nurse must be aware of the functioning of the organisation as a whole and the potential struggles within it. Only with an understanding of the whole picture can the nurse hope to provide support to the patient as it becomes the product of interaction and relationships with the multi-professional team rather than a simple relationship between nurse and patient.

The Nursing and Midwifery Council (NMC, 2008: 3) include membership of multi-disciplinary teams as one of their standards of proficiency saying that nurses must: 'Work cooperatively within teams and respect the skills, expertise and contributions of colleagues.' The nurse can lead or follow depending what is needed for that person at that time.

Senior nurses, as Arnold et al. (2006) point out, must engage with a different range of professionals, such as managers and finance directors, in order to ensure that patients receive proper and ethical care. At this level, nurses must engage with the entire management structure of the organisation to ensure that there is equitable distribution of resources both for patients and for the nursing team for whom they are responsible.

Ellis et al. (2005: 276) see another role for nurses within the team. They suggest that it is the nurse who filters the vast amount of information coming from many different health professionals, in order to provide a coherent picture for patients and their families.

The pattern of health care delivery is constantly changing and one of the features to have developed over recent years is nurse-led care. Nurses are taking the lead in innovative schemes, from rehabilitation to emergency care. These schemes may be designed to promote cost effectiveness or improve patient outcomes. They might relieve pressure on the medical team, reduce pressure on other facilities as, for instance, NHS walk-in centres are designed to do or might lead because the nurse's holistic approach best suits the situation. These new roles develop as a result of negotiation between professional groups as well as government policy makers and patient groups as all must support these changing professional boundaries if these innovations are to be successful (Chapple et al., 2000). Rick Fisher explores these new roles in more detail in the next chapter.

Nurses have proven ability as effective leaders in these areas but they still struggle to take the leadership roles that shape the wider development of health care. Kitson (2004) urges nurses to shed the 'constraining myths and stereotypes' that limit the profession's ability to contribute to health care transformation.

The nurse as specialist

Some of the therapist roles with which we are now so familiar, such as physiotherapy, have emerged from a group of nurses who saw a need to specialise (www.csp.org. uk/director/about/thecsp/history.cfm), but the very flexibility that makes nursing so hard to define is its central feature. In more recent times nurses have specialised in ever-increasing areas but have retained their status of nurse. These specialities might be related to specific diseases such as diabetes or Parkinson's disease; to systems such as heart or renal systems or to techniques such as endoscopy or in specialist areas such as emergency care practice or rehabilitation of older people. Specialist nurses often work particularly closely with doctors and may be empowered to become involved in diagnosis and prescription of medication within their speciality. Their relationship with other professional groups may be altered by their authority to make direct referrals. Groups such as physiotherapists and radiographers must have the confidence that these nurses are sufficiently skilled to request their input as, traditionally, only doctors would have done.

Nurses bring their own fundamental professional values and framework and may take a different approach, spending more time on education or supportive activities. Spilsbury and Meyer (2001: 9) point out that it is impossible to assume that nurses taking over the role of doctors will be more cost effective as 'it cannot be presumed that nurses substituting for doctors will provide care in the same way as doctors.'

Having spent some time defining nursing and exploring the role of the nurse, the following case study develops your reading further. The case study is based on the needs of Mr G and has several purposes. First, it sets out some of the multi-professional roles and relationships the nurse may have as he or she supports Mr G. It also highlights in more detail the professional role and function of the nurse in practice. Significantly it illustrates where all of these liaisons and interventions are centred – on the needs of Mr G and the relationship the nurse negotiates and builds with him.

Case study: Mr G

Mr G, a retired school teacher from Northern Ireland, is 79-years-old and has smoked 20 cigarettes a day all his adult life. His practice nurse discussed his general health when he came for a blood pressure check – he has been taking medication for hypertension for several years. Despite the medication, Mr G's blood pressure is higher than when last checked. The nurse asks Mr G about his lifestyle and finds that he has a high consumption of processed food since his wife died three months ago. He explains that his wife did all the cooking and he doesn't know much about making healthy meals. The nurse tells Mr G that the community dietician runs classes about healthy eating and offers to refer Mr G. She also tells him about a local luncheon club where he could buy a cooked meal twice a week and make new friends. Knowing that Mr G smokes, she asks if he would like her to discuss the possibility of using nicotine patches with the doctor. She has suggested these before and Mr G was not keen but he does now feel that he should 'give it a go'.

Nurses do not view their role as restricted to those who are currently sick but see recipients of nursing care as including healthy people and those who are at risk of developing disease (Zarzycka and Slusarska, 2007). A focus on promoting health and helping individuals, families and groups to meet their health needs is seen by the QAA as a key feature of nursing (QAA, 2001). Health promotion, according to Orme et al. (2007) takes a distinctive multi-professional perspective on health. Many different professional groups have an important part to play. Occupational therapists can provide equipment and home adaptations that can prevent falls; physiotherapists can tailor exercise programmes to individual needs – but to use their skills these professionals have to know that there is a risk to health and may rely on the nurse to direct people to their services.

In this case the nurse needs to discuss some issues with other professionals.

Guided Study 2.1

What would the nurse need to know to access other support services and professionals to help Mr G with his attempt to quit smoking and dietary needs?

You could have included:

Knowing what is available requires not only understanding of the expert skills of the multi-professional team, but also a good knowledge of the structure of the local health and third sector services as they may vary from district to district.

Mr. G could self-refer to the group run by the dietician but would not have done so if the nurse had not provided the information and encouragement. To practice effectively the nurse must have an extensive network of contacts so that appropriate health promotion interventions can be initiated. The nurse is also relying on a good relationship with Mr G. It is only because he has come to her that he has overcome his reticence to try interventions such as nicotine patches and accept referral to other professionals.

The nurse is concerned that Mr G is not coping well with the death of his wife. She asks him if he would like her to chat to the GP about services that might help him. The GP is the gatekeeper who must make the actual referral to bereavement counselling services but, without the nurse's awareness of the role that counsellors play, the doctor would not have been alerted to the need.

The nurse routinely gives her patients a leaflet describing the role of service users in shaping and evaluating care provision and facilities. Mr G decides that he would like to use his experience to help others so he rings the number on the leaflet and volunteers to become the user representative at his local Antrim Area Hospital. He becomes involved in the group and enjoys the sense of making a worthwhile contribution to his local community – he feels that his past career as a teacher makes him well suited to speaking up on behalf of others. He finds that all members of the interdisciplinary team really are interested in listening to his experiences both as a patient and as a carer during his wife's illness.

Mr G takes up all the health promotion opportunities suggested and continues to live a simple but satisfying life for several years. Now aged 85, he wakes up one day from his after-dinner nap to find that one side of his body feels heavy and strange. As he tries to stand up he finds that his limbs on that side are not responding properly. Alarmed, he rings NHS Direct and speaks to a nurse. Her assessment is that of probable stroke and that immediate hospital treatment is needed. She alerts the ambulance service, efficiently giving them the information they need in order to prioritise the case. Mr G is rushed to hospital. In the emergency department a nurse meets Mr G. who is being transferred from the ambulance. Paramedics give a brief handover explaining how their assessment using FAST has led them to support stroke as the cause of Mr G's collapse and explaining what treatments they have given on route to the hospital.

Box 2.1 Stroke Symptom Recognition

Recognising stroke symptoms using **FAST**

- **F**acial weakness
- **A**rm and leg weakness
- **S**peech problems
- **T**est these signs.

These two professional groups share a language and understanding that allows for total continuity of care. Departmental and national protocols demand that stroke is treated as an emergency (DoH, 2001c) with the administration of thrombolytic medication where appropriate. The nurse knows that this must be done within a three-hour window (Woodford, 2007) if damage to brain tissue is to be minimised, but that first there must be certain that this stroke is the result of an embolus and not a bleed. Giving thrombolytic medication to the smaller number of patients who have actually suffered an intercranial haemorrhage could increase bleeding with potentially disastrous effect. The nurse cannot act alone. It is the doctor who will make the final decisions but gathering information and setting the process in motion will save valuable time and greatly improve Mr G's chances of survival. The nurse asks the medical technician to take routine observations and establish an intravenous line while she contacts the doctor and alerts the duty radiographer to the fact that a brain scan will be needed.

Despite life saving treatment from the emergency team, Mr G shows signs of residual brain damage. The emergency department nurse hands over his care to a nursing colleague on the stroke assessment unit. This stroke assessment unit is set up as a blending point for various professional groups – many of whom are actually based within the unit so contributing to a very close working relationship in the multi-professional team. Shared records are used so that each professional group knows exactly what is being done by the others and what the various different professional assessments have revealed. The traditional nursing handover is replaced by a daily team meeting in which all professional groups come together to discuss plans and progress.

The speech and language therapist will assess swallowing and Mr G must remain 'nil by mouth' until this is done (Paciaroni et al., 2004). Over the next few weeks food and fluids will be reintroduced as the therapist deems that it is safe to do so. The dietician will ensure that food provided includes the necessary nutrients and is of the right consistency. But it is the nurse who has the final responsibility of ensuring that Mr G is well positioned and closely supervised so that he can safely eat.

The physiotherapist will be involved from an early stage to ensure that movements and positions minimise deformity and enhance balance. Mr G will have therapy sessions in the gym but, in between sessions, therapeutic positioning and exercise must be maintained; this is the role of the nurse. Throughout the 24-hour period nurses will closely follow the physiotherapist's plan. Without this continuity the impact of the isolated therapy sessions would be greatly reduced. This would mean, not only that Mr G's recovery would be slower but also that he might never regain the function that he could in the care of a well integrated multi-professional team.

The occupational therapist assesses the particular ways in which brain damage has altered function and advises on programmes to maximise functional potential. A speech and language therapist is involved again to help Mr G regain some control in losses in speech. The clinical psychologist explores ways of helping Mr G and his family cope with his altered body image and loss of function. While the doctor is acknowledged as team leader in this unit, it is the nurse who is at the hub of inter-disciplinary activity. The need for those intimate and caring skills is high and, at the same time, the 24-hour presence of the nursing team means that only they can ensure that the regimes planned by other team members are enacted; further, they ensure that the multi-professional team's records are maintained in a way that allows the different members to act in harmony, and to keep a constant watchful eye, ready to call appropriate professional help if the situation changes or to act as stopgap if they are not available. The nurse is also best placed to develop a relationship with Mr G's family, who will be vital to a successful discharge.

Guided Study 2.2

In the case study above a number of professional roles are presented. Describe these roles and their function in the multi-professional team.

Mr G makes good progress and is discharged home with the support of a multi-professional intermediate care team. Membership of intermediate care teams varies according to local decisions. In this case the core members are:

- Physiotherapist
- Occupational therapist
- Social worker
- Nurse specialist
- Rehabilitation care assistant.

The team has also negotiated special fast referral routes to:

- District nurse
- Community psychiatric nurse
- Speech and language specialist
- Consultant geriatrician
- Psychologist
- Dietician
- Pharmacist
- Care and repair/handy man
- Home economist
- Voluntary services coordinator.

Here the nursing role is less central but still important, providing the first point of contact for emotional support and a link with the GP and the rest of the primary care team.

Mr G progresses well for a few months but then increasing frailty leads his family to seek a residential care placement. Assessments are made by a new multi-professional team. Now the main player becomes the social worker, who works with an NHS nurse to establish the level of need, the most appropriate care package and the level of financial support that Mr G is entitled to. After consultation, Mr G is admitted to Riverview care home, which provides 24-hour nursing support. The nurses here liaise most closely with the GP and the pharmacist at the local high street chemist. The home has regular visits from a physiotherapist, a podiatrist and a music therapist. Additional charges are made for these services so nurses discuss the available options with Mr G and his family and then discuss their requests with the visiting professionals.

Six months later Mr G is found unconscious in his room. A nursing support worker presses the alarm to summon the nurse, who calls the ambulance and explains the situation to the paramedics who arrive on the scene. The cycle begins again except that this time the prognosis is poor. Mr G is admitted to a palliative care ward. Here the nurse practices at the centre of a very different multi-professional team. He or she liaises with the doctor and hospital pharmacist and also with the hospital chaplain and the bereavement coordinator, who can offer support to the family in the coming months.

In the various stages of Mr G's journey, different professionals have taken the lead in care. The nurse's role in relation to these professional groups has changed as the situation has changed but has very often provided a communication link between professional groups or between the professional and Mr G and his family. As well as being the provider of both intimate and highly technical care, it is the nurse who has translated the regimes planned by other professionals into 24-hour care and has been the eyes and ears ready to alert the team to any change. Without the pivotal and flexible role of the nurse the team could not have functioned.

Guided Study 2.3

We can see the importance of the nurse's role in ensuring people get the best care whatever their health and social care needs. The key to this is multi-professional liaison and collaboration. Think about your experience in practice so far. What types of activity have you seen nurses undertake and what skills have they used?

Need to know more?

These website links will help you:
www.nmc-uk.org
www.rcn.org.uk
www.nhscareers.nhs.uk/nursing.shtml

Conclusion

Multi-professional practice is a dynamic entity. It is constantly shaped by newly emerging professional groups, such as medical assistants; by changing roles within existing medical groups; by organisational changes at local and national level and by advances in knowledge and technology. The nurse needs to keep abreast of these changes so that he or she can continue to work in a way that best meets patients' needs.

The multi-professional health team comes in many guises. Both the make-up and the leadership of the team vary according to the situation. The part played by nurses is equally variable. To function best in the multi-professional arena, the nurse must be confident of those caring elements that define nursing and must also have the knowledge, flexibility and communication skills that aid the functioning of the whole team.

3

Multi-professional Practice in Primary Care Nursing
Rick Fisher

By reading this chapter you should be able to:

- **identify legislative drivers for changes in the multi-professional team in primary care**
- **describe new and emerging roles for the nurse in the multi-professional team in primary care**
- **begin to develop a definition of community**
- **undertake a preliminary community assessment to review the fit and capacity of available services**
- **consider changes in the community and their impact on service delivery**
- **access websites to find out more about demographic changes in the community**
- **unify this learning to put in place a plan to facilitate your personal development needs for multi-professional working.**

Introduction

As society changes and notions of what constitutes a 'community' alter, primary care services need to realign themselves to meet different needs and expectations from the public. Primary care itself is undergoing major transformation, which raises a new set of challenges for those working in the field. In this chapter the legislative frameworks in place to drive change are presented, and multi-professional working is investigated from three key perspectives. Initially the changing role of the nurse in response to service redesign, as a re-negotiation of professional boundaries and emerging new positions takes place. Second, the impact of changing communities on multi-professional working and its components and, finally, drawing on your personal experience to consider how equipped you are as a nurse to operate in this new world of practice.

Legislative and policy framework

The NHS Plan: A Plan for Investment, A Plan for Reform (DoH, 2000) set out a ten-year programme of investment and reform by the government. The main objective of the plan is to provide a 'NHS fit for the 21st century', setting out a framework of standards, accountability, devolution of power and resources designed to free professionals who deliver care from existing constraints, in order for them to innovate and provide 'increased flexibility between services and between staff to cut across outdated organisational and professional barriers' (DoH, 2002a: 8). It also emphasised the need for patients, whom it called consumers, to have greater choice, which would be provided by an increase in the diversity of providers of health care. The key message underpinning this legislation was an objective to liberate the talents and skills of the entire workforce 'so that every patient gets the right care in the right place at the right time' (DoH, 2002a: 34).

Within all of the recent health care legislation is the undeniable shift in the centre of power which has turned the NHS on its head. For the first time since its inception in 1948, the health service is to be driven by primary care, which is care given outside of institutions in the Acute Sector. The Department of Health describes *primary* care as community based health services that are usually the first, and often the only, point of contact that patients make with the health service. It covers services provided by family doctors (GPs), community and practice nurses, community therapists (such as physiotherapists and occupational therapists), community pharmacists, optometrists, dentists and midwives (www.dh.gov.uk/en/Aboutus/HowDHworks/DH_074639 accessed November 20th 2007).

This change of emphasis means power and responsibility for the delivery and purchase of *all* health care being devolved from the centralised Department of Health through Strategic Health Authorities to Primary Care Trusts (PCTs). Simultaneously the publication of *Shifting the Balance of Power: The Next Steps* (DoH, 2002b) placed the emphasis on to the patient, who was to become central to all processes, but also included 'frontline' health care staff in the decision-making activity. It was less prescriptive than many previous government documents, explicitly enabling decisions to be taken locally, according to the needs of the population. Crucially, it noted that such radical proposals would need to invoke radical responses from all concerned and the paper stressed the need to change traditional behaviours of professionals in their approach to roles. Chief Executive Nigel Crisp noted, in particular, the need for a shift in culture that was required in order for the reforms to take place.

Table 3.1   A Shift in Culture

	From	To
A shift in organisation and ways of working	• Hierarchical and nationalised Detailed guidance with many milestones and targets • Focus on institutions	• Devolved local networks • Clear long term outcomes with latitude about method • Working through networks
A shift in the scale and quality of staff, patient and community involvement	• Small pockets of excellence • Many enthusiasts but not fully embedded • Supported by 'time limited' soft funding • Many Boards still viewing this as peripheral to core business	• Mainstream way of achieving change • Professional and systematic everywhere • Properly resourced through recurring funds • Central to Boards' way of working
A shift in management focus	• All management effort driven by delivery of centrally imposed key targets as ends in themselves • Meetings, plans and strategy dominating management time • Risk avoidance because of fear of penalties	• Delivery of targets achieved as the by-product of wider and sustained improvements in service quality • Walking the job with a strong focus on clinical quality • Incentives as a key part of improvement • Penalties seen by all as fair

Source: Shifting Balance of Power: The Next Steps (DoH, 2002b)

New and emerging models of service delivery in primary care

To put in place these new and more flexible services, legislation has been designed to free up PCTs to tender for and commission them. The White Paper *Our Health, Our Care, Our Say* (DoH, 2006b), based on offering more individualised and user friendly care, is the driver for these changes in service models, while *Fairness in Primary Care* (DoH, 2007e) is a procurement model to enable commissioners of care to tender and purchase them in areas where inequality of service is present. New strategies for developing and funding these services are in place, notably NHSLIFT (DoH, 2007f), which enables private and public sector services to work together to offer radically different options for patients or service users. One example of this are walk-in centres, which were designed in part to alleviate the workload placed on accident and emergency departments, who were becoming inundated with inappropriate self-referrals. These frequently occurred because many people were unable to contact their GP out of hours, or were not registered with a GP. Walk-in centres operate from convenient sites, including high streets and, in at least one case, railway stations. They operate seven days a week; mostly from 7am until 10pm. Services they offer include a consultation with an experienced NHS nurse, treatment for minor injuries and illnesses, health advice and information on other local services.

New care delivery plans also include the franchising of GP services, while there are developing partnerships between commercial industry and the Department of Health. In 2005, Boots the Chemist entered a joint agreement with the Department of Health to provide chlamydia screening in 201 high street stores. This broke with tradition, as any person who wished to be screened could approach the service without the need for a referral from a medical practitioner.

The government has recently set out further endorsement of the role of primary care in its review of the NHS. The document *High Quality Care For All* (DoH, 2008b) includes plans to continue the commissioning role of the PCT. There will be increased partnerships with the third sector and further development of the personalised care service model and emphasis on increased choice. As PCTs gain in importance their role as employers of nurses will gain increasing momentum. For nurses in primary care this is likely to have the following implications.

Box 3.1   Implications of Primary Care-driven NHS on Nurses:

- A service where patients and the public have a greater choice and a greater voice
- Opportunities to provide more secondary care in community settings
- Extending nursing roles, including taking on some work currently done by GPs
- A key role in delivering 24-hour first contact care across a range of settings
- A major role in delivering National Service Frameworks
- Having a greater voice in decision making
- A focus on prevention and tackling inequalities
- Greater skill mix and leadership opportunities.

(*Liberating the Talents*, DoH, 2002c)

Within *Liberating the Talents: Helping Primary Care Trusts and Nurses to Deliver the NHS Plan* (DoH, 2002c) was a clear statement that there would be a commitment to 'extending nursing roles including taking on some work currently done by GPs', which was further endorsed by including nurse prescribing as one of the ten key roles for nurses. Autonomy was effectively increased in the same part of this document with the statement that nurses would be required to take the lead in the way local health services are organised and the way that they are run. Additionally, *Liberating the Talents* made reference to how the new General Medical Services contract would create more opportunities for flexible working to meet the needs of patients, closer cross-practice and PCT joint working. In tandem with this the Chief Nursing Officer for England (CNO) set out ten key roles for nurses within the NHS modernisation agenda.

Box 3.2   The Chief Nursing Officer's Ten Key Roles for Nurses

- To order diagnostic investigations such as pathology test and x-rays
- To make and receive referrals directly, say, to a therapist or a pain consultant
- To admit and discharge patients for specified conditions and within agreed protocols
- To manage patient caseloads, say, for diabetes or rheumatology
- To run clinics, say, for ophthalmology or dermatology
- To prescribe medicines and treatments
- To carry out a wide range of resuscitation procedures including defibrillation
- To perform minor surgery and outpatient procedures
- To triage patients using the latest IT to the most appropriate health professional
- To take the lead in the way local health services are organised and the way that they are run.

An additional piece of legislation which is having considerable impact upon the ways professionals will operate and, indeed, how they will collaborate, is that introduced under the banner of the *NHS Knowledge and Skills Framework (KSF)* which was introduced in October 2004 (DoH, 2004a). The Framework 'defines and describes the knowledge and skills which NHS staff need to apply in their work in order to deliver quality services'. It provides 'a single, consistent, comprehensive and explicit framework on which to base review and development for all staff' (2004a: 3). The above statement is slightly misleading, because doctors, dentists and some senior NHS Managers are exempted from the KSF. However, it is linked to the all important *Agenda for Change* (DoH, 2004b) and as such is a crucial element in linking activity and performance with salary. Therefore, it is possible to see exactly how an individual member of staff, taking into consideration the freedom offered by the legislation, can participate in care delivery in a less restricted manner.

This might be interpreted as enabling legislation which will empower professionals from all backgrounds to undertake any task which they feel – and can demonstrate competence in – equipped to perform. The implication for multi-professional working is that fewer areas of caring will be the domain of a single profession. This has become evident with the evolving roles being undertaken by a variety of professionals in recent years. Pharmacists, along with other Allied Health Professionals (AHPs) such as physiotherapists and occupational therapists, can join nurses in undertaking education in order to become prescribers. Nurses working in walk-in centres can order a variety of investigations and treatments, which were until recently the exclusive province of medical practitioners, in their own professional right. Nurses in primary care collaborating with professionals in older people services may be meeting with them in new and emerging services based on social entrepreneurship. Within this type of model businesses work to offer social care to promote positive practices, and may enter into partnerships between business agencies and practitioners.

With this expansion and blurring of roles, as described in *Liberating the Talents: Helping Primary Care Trusts and Nurses to Deliver the NHS Plan* (DoH, 2002c), comes a requirement for all involved to collaborate in ways which ensure both the safety and centrality of the patient. Some examples of these new approaches for nursing practice are now discussed.

Nurse prescribing

Following a lengthy campaign initiated by the Cumberlege Report (Neighbourhood Nursing – A Focus For Care 1986) nurse prescribing was introduced in England and Wales in 2000. The enabling legislation, the Medicinal Products: Prescription by Nurses Act (DoH, 1992b) was a radical departure from the traditional approach to prescribing which until this time had been the sole province of medical practitioners. In its current guise, nurse prescribing is evolving rapidly. Initially it was restricted to District Nurses and Health Visitors, but has been expanded to include all first level registered nurses who have undertaken specific educational programmes to prepare them for the role of prescriber. The educational process has necessarily required multi-professional collaboration in its instigation, involving pharmacy lecturers, medical practitioners and legal advisors. In the practice setting prescribing is based on multi-professional collaboration between designated nurses, doctors and pharmacists who work together with patients and carers to ensure that prescribed materials are delivered appropriately and efficiently. For example, where patients have difficulty in taking prescribed medications from complicated prescriptions, doctors, pharmacists and community nurses collaborate to organise a system such as the use of Dosset boxes or blister packs of medication, based on the nursing assessment of their ability to self administer the regime.

Deciding when resuscitation should take place

The most recent example of a non-traditional approach to multi-professional working – at the time of writing – is the joint statement by the Royal College of Nursing (RCN), the Resuscitation Council (UK) and the British Medical Association (BMA) regarding cardio-pulmonary resuscitation (CPR). This document addresses a very complex situation regarding the emotive subject of when to decide whether CPR should be attempted. The Do Not Attempt Resuscitation (DNAR) document (2007) states:

> The overall clinical responsibility for decisions about CPR, including DNAR decisions, rests with the most senior clinician in charge of the patient's care as defined by local policy. This could be a consultant, GP or suitably experienced nurse. He or she should always be prepared to discuss a CPR decision for any individual patient with other health professionals involved in the patient's care. Teamwork and good communication are of paramount importance. (BMA, Resuscitation Council (UK, RCN, 2007: 19)

This innovation represents a departure from previous practice in which such decisions were in the domain of medical practitioners alone. The collaboration of the three organisations to create these guidelines is a clear example of the ways in which multi-professional working is having an effect on the ways in which members of these professions work together. Although it is far too early to assess the impact of this new approach it is possible to anticipate that relationships between the professionals involved should improve when there is a clear demonstration of collaboration in the leadership of all the professions involved.

National Dementia Strategy

The National Dementia Strategy, announced in August 2007, aims to address the rising number of cases of dementias that are occurring. Recognising that the number of people suffering from dementia will double in the next 30 years, the government has acknowledged that the existing system is not adequate to meet expanding needs. The Strategy is designed to bring together a stakeholder group comprising representatives of the Alzheimer's Society, Age Concern, Help the Aged, the Royal College of Nursing and the Royal College of Psychiatrists. By the summer of 2008 Ministers will announce a transformation plan to ensure dementia services are improved in all parts of the country. Another clear example of an attempt to place the service user at the centre of the service. Representatives of users' organisations will be clearly involved from the outset of this initiative. In order for this strategy to be effective all organisations from the statutory, charitable and voluntary sectors will need to collaborate in effective partnerships.

Intermediate care

Intermediate care is a central element of the government's modernisation agenda. It has been developed to promote speedier recovery from illness, prevent unnecessary acute hospital admission, support timely discharge and maximise independent living. Utilising a range of integrated services it is a prime example of how professionals from a variety of disciplines can work together to provide a seamless care delivery system. Its aim is to 'enhance appropriateness and quality of care for individuals' (DoH, 2002d) and in the process will make a significant impact on the health and social care system as a whole by making more effective use of capacity and establishing new ways of working. Intermediate care can be seen as an important factor in implementing the National Service Framework for Older People. However, all four countries of the United Kingdom use different definitions of what it entails. The NHS Information Centre, illustrates this with its document 'Short definitions of Intermediate Care' (www.ic. nhs.uk, accessed 26 February 2008). Regardless of this confusion with terminology and importantly in the context of this book, intermediate care necessarily relies on multi-professional working, because it involves many different professionals from a variety of organisations and sectors. These include health and social care professionals and representatives from organisations such as local authorities or other agencies involved in providing housing, for example charitable housing trusts. Voluntary organisations also play a major part in contributing to the holistic approach. For example, the Women's Royal Voluntary Service is still the largest single provider of 'meals on wheels' in the United Kingdom (DoH, 2005). In Chapter 9 Terry Scragg explores the role of the third sector in more detail.

Case study: 'Ruby'

Ruby is 82-years-old. She has lived independently for many years having been widowed at the age of 40. Ruby, who suffers from arthritis, retired to the coast, retiring from her job as a clerical officer in the civil service. In recent years she has become more forgetful and her usually meticulous record keeping has become more erratic, as has her ability to maintain her personal hygiene and culinary skills. This deterioration in her physical and mental health has contributed to several incidents where she has forgotten to pay her bills, and resulted in embarrassing scenes in the local newsagent. The general practitioner referred Ruby to the local Day Centre. Here she is able to participate in reminiscence therapy with the community mental health nursing team; the social worker has helped address some of the financial concerns raised by her diminishing mental capacity and the consultant in rheumatology has been able to assess her needs as her arthritis progresses. An Occupational Therapist has arranged for an assessment of her home environment while the District Nurse acts as the Key Worker who coordinates all of these services. This example illustrates how properly coordinated multi-professional collaboration can enhance the quality of life for people, enabling them to maintain their dignity and remain in their own homes with minimal intervention.

Gaps in the legislation

The above legislatory frameworks assume that all are working for the good of patients and service users as their primary aim. They do not, however, acknowledge the power relationships that exist between the various players, both as individuals and as members of professional bodies. Neither do they recognise the real power of professional closure, for example when professionals deliberately hold on to information to maintain dominance over the case regardless of the potential impact on the patient or service user. When exercised this activity has the potential to prevent true collaboration. You have already seen that roles are changing and boundaries are being blurred. This can create stress and role conflict for some professionals who may have previously ensured that there was a claim to some exclusive role. For doctors in particular, this may be a threat, as they have seen both diagnosis and treatment, in the form of limited prescribing, removed from their exclusive domain.

Tovey and Adams (2001) talk about the constant review of general practitioners roles, with an emphasis on 'responsibilities, independence, status and authority', noting the tension between autonomy and accountability. They discuss the increasing influence of and emphasis on public and lay involvement in health care delivery in the community and the tension between professional self-interest and managerial (service) demands. A tension exists, when challenges are made regarding the right of professionals to exercise autonomy, in the interests of patients.

This is amplified by Peckham and Exworthy (2003), who note that with the introduction of new professions, such as complementary therapists, and with the blurring of boundaries between lay people and professionals, there is a 'changing balance of power between professionals, tensions between professional groups and the organizational structure within which professionals work' (2003: 159).

So although there is a degree of consensus that – in the interests of the patient or service user – multi-professional working is an admirable concept, there may be limitations to both professional will and legislation, which mean that such collaborative working is not yet at the centre of practice that governments clearly desire it to be. However, progress is being made towards this goal and the following sections shows how this is taking place.

Proactive approaches to partnership working

For nurses to succeed in the modern NHS and indeed within any health care agency – be they statutory or voluntary in nature – it is not sufficient to remain reactive to change. Successful partners will adopt a proactive approach which will enable them to become key participants in multi-professional care provision. This may be achieved by developing an approach to caring which undertakes holistic assessment that is far wider than has previously been the case. It may encompass a community-wide assessment to gain a working knowledge of agencies which can be approached to collaborate in care within a specified geographical region. Those of you who have had experience in a Community Nursing arena will be familiar with a Community Needs Assessment, while for others this will be a new and exciting development of your practice. Before considering assessment it is necessary to examine the notion of 'community'.

'Community' is a slippery concept; it can mean different things to different people and it is evident that this can be problematic. Jones (1994) reflected that although the term 'community' was in common use by members of the caring professions and politicians, each of these professions has their own interpretation of what it should mean. Jones further notes that the use and interpretation of the term by these professionals is not constant. Community does, however, consist of a number of characteristics which enable it to be defined in a more satisfactory manner. These characteristics or dimensions, according to Orr (1992) can be considered under the following four headings.

The community as a locality

This refers to the geographical boundaries of the community. Some may consider this to be the easiest concept to grasp as it has a physical property. It could readily be aligned with entities such as a town, a village, an electoral ward or a housing estate. However, this approach to community is rather simplistic because it tells us very little other than the physical properties of the community.

The community as social structure

This involves the cansideration of the people who live within the community, with particular emphasis on their social characteristics. These will include their demographic details such as age, gender, ethnicity and their employment status.

Social activity

This describes what actually happens in the community, encompassing the facilities and resources which are available to the people within the community.

Community as sentiment

This takes note of the way it feels to live in a particular place. What are the positive and negative aspects of living in an area; do people have pride in their homes; are the shops and public buildings clean and pleasant, or does the area appear to be deprived? How do people who don't live in the area feel about the area?

Assessing the community

Assessment of a community depends on the formulation of a community profile. Tinson (1995) explains that a nurse seeking to understand a community will need, in the first instance, to define the boundaries of that community. Her example (1995: 159) considers that different professionals will define the boundaries according to their speciality. For district nurses, this may consist of a particular general practice population, while for health visitors it may be the electoral ward; school nurses may confine their community to one school or expand it to a group of schools. However, this process may become even more complex as services merge and trusts develop new spheres as new integrated design, planning and delivery of services takes place and boundaries for practice become less clear.

Having carefully identified the structures in which he or she practises, the nurse will need to undertake a profile of the community that has been defined. Hawtin et al. (1994: 5) define a community profile as:

A comprehensive description of the needs of a population that is defined, or defines itself, as a community, and the resources that exist within that community, carried out with the active involvement of the community itself, for the purpose of developing an action plan or other means of improving the quality of life within the community.

Having gathered the data which will form the profile, professionals can prioritise the need which exists in that community, in order to improve services within it. As Hawtin et al. explain above, members of the community are involved in the process and the important aspect of the profile and thereafter the assessment, is that it is not solely driven by the perceptions of the professionals. In this way it is possible to produce an assessment which reflects the perspectives of all of those who will be involved, both users and providers of services.

Guided Study 3.1

What is a community wide assessment?
Consider the area in which you are currently working or living.

Ask yourself:

- Can I identify this area as a 'community'?
- What characteristics can I identify about this 'community' using the headings:
  - The community as a locality
  - The community as a social structure
  - The community as a social activity
  - The community as a sentiment.

Need to know more?

The following websites might help:
If you have time you might want to look at other national demographic indicators and how they may be changing, such as the Office for National Statistics, which can provide information on your postcode area, see: neighbourhood.statistics.gov.uk/dissemination/ Or for information on birth rates and death rates in the area see www.gro.gov.uk/gro/content/

Having achieved this, consider whether the services that exist in the community adequately meet the needs of the people who live there. Use available evidence to support your findings.

- Have you identified any gaps in provision for the community?
- If so, how might these be addressed?

- Are new models of service delivery being introduced?
- If there are no gaps, how might existing provision be improved?
- What factors might impact on provision levels in the community?

The preceding section of this chapter should help you to identify the various character-istics of your community. You will recognise that what you have discovered is your indi-vidual perception and you may wish to discuss this with a colleague, preferably one from a different profession to your own, or a lay member of the community.

Negotiating boundaries for partnership working

One of the major hurdles to be overcome when attempting partnership working is that of negotiating boundaries. This is vitally important if resources are to be used efficiently and effectively. For the service user and the professionals involved, it is also of para-mount importance to ensure that errors of repetition and/or omission do not occur. This can be achieved by the acknowledgement, as stated previously in this chapter, that boundaries do exist between the various people or services in the system. For this rea-son, whenever an individual episode of complex care is being planned, all those who are to be involved in the care process must be included at the planning stage. Boundaries, of what is practicable and more importantly, what is acceptable, must be negotiated.

Acceptability is perhaps a fluid concept, for the attitudes of professionals and service users can change over time, even during the same episode of care. Similarly, needs and capabilities may change over a period of time. Brooks and Brown (2002) illustrate this. They observe the ceremonial aspect of care giving, based on the 'who does what' approach. They also recognise that if care is to become more flexible and suited to indi-viduals, at times professionals will need to adapt their approach to care delivery. This results in a comment on the strategies which may have been used to eradicate cere-monies which reinforce the status quo within an organisation, while at the same time encourage the adoption of new ceremonies to promote changes. Naming these as 'Ceremonies of Preservation' and 'Ceremonies of Change', respectively, Brooks and Brown noted that within the former there was a tendency for tasks to be repeated when separate professional groups were involved. This was particularly apparent in the recording of patient details, which became repetitive. Within the ceremonies of change was the attempt to produce 'patient-centred' care wherein cross-professional collabora-tion is legitimised by placing emphasis on the patient rather than the professional. This attempt at initiating change should not be taken only at face value, for it is also provid-ing a challenge to the cultural mechanisms and tribal thinking which exists within the health care organisation. Within the account is a continued reference to legitimisation of change. For example, clinical protocols may require that a district nurse engages a general practitioner to undertake a rectal examination to assess a patient before a deci-sion can be made regarding the use of an enema. Supplying the doctor with the neces-sary equipment to administer an enema, which he/she can give at the time of the examination, reduces distress and gives immediate care for the patient while reducing the workload for the whole team. Such a practice is outside the conventional model, but, by renegotiating the 'who does what' boundaries, it is possible to provide a seamless approach to care. It is, therefore, essential that some form of plan be negotiated, in which all participants in care and most importantly, the service user, are agreed on the boundaries which have been discussed. The plan should be signed by all participants, with stated review dates in order to monitor its effectiveness.

Guided Study 3.2

In your practice have you noticed any ceremonies of preservation or change occurring? Why do you think they occur and for whose benefit?
What needs to change for these to stop?
What inter- or multi-professional skills and knowledge are required to make changes happen?

You could have included:
Ceremonies of preservation:
Routine tasks being left until the 'right' person is available to do them
Activities being undertaken in a certain way 'because we've always done it this way'
Activities being undertaken because the method or 'routine' suits the professionals involved.
Ceremonies of change:
Attempts, whether successful or not, to change something in order to make life better for the service user.

Need to know more?

Did you discuss how the professionals you worked with might like to change certain activities?
Did you identify education and/or training that might be required, for example joint training on partnerships with service users?
Make a note to explore this with your practice supervisor next time you meet with her.

Flexible approaches to roles and practices linked to potential new multi-professional roles for nurses

Nursing has evolved and is continuing to do so at a breathtaking pace. Nurses have extended their professional repertoire to include diagnosis and treatment of a variety of conditions, becoming key specialists in areas such as the management of diabetes and tissue viability. In the future, nurses will be required to further expand their approach to working collaboratively with and for patients in a variety of settings. Roles such as that of the Community Matron, which include diagnosing, prescribing, treating and evaluating the care of patients, will become more commonplace. Guidance for these developing roles and the potential for further expansions can be found if you return to the CNO's ten key roles for nurses. You should bear these in mind when considering your future role as a nurse or when negotiating your developmental needs at your meeting with your supervisor.

Guided Study 3.3

First of all reflect on how the information you have gained from reading this book so far might impact on your approach to multi-professional working.
Next think about your future role as a qualified nurse.

Undertake a SWOT analysis in which you focus primarily on the multi-professional aspect of your work.

A SWOT analysis is a method of examining the Strengths, Weaknesses, Opportunities and Threats which present themselves to an organisation. This approach began in the Harvard Business School in the 1950s and is still widely used. An individual can also use these categories to examine where he or she excels, and also address areas which need to be improved on in order to reach their maximum potential. As a student nurse you may wish to consider a SWOT analysis by asking these questions in the following manner:

Strengths	which aspects of my professional life are most successful?
Weaknesses	which are the areas where I need to make improvements?
Opportunities	where can I gain help or information which will help me to make the improvements? Which opportunities will help me to use my strengths to the greatest advantage?
Threats	what are the factors which might make it difficult for me to improve my practice?

If you have identified that your strengths lie in your ability to communicate with others, yet you have a weakness in your current clinical skills, you may take the opportunity to practise these skills with help from a more experienced practitioner. A threat may occur if you are reluctant to seek advice or help to improve your situation.

Guided Study 3.4

Take some time to reflect on your current working situation and examine your performance using the SWOT analysis as explained above.
Think about the results of your SWOT analysis. What have you learned?

By identifying your strengths you should be able to demonstrate which aspects of your professional role you consider you are most competent in. Similarly, identifying your weaknesses will highlight areas in which you feel you are less able. Examining the opportunities that exist will help you to become equipped to develop your own skills in order to enhance your ability to work in a multi-professional role. This might include formal and/or informal education which will equip you to work in a multi-professional environment. Finally, you should examine areas which might be considered threats to your own development. These might be sub-divided into *intrinsic* and *extrinsic* threats. For the former, these could include your own attitude to members of other professions, perhaps based on previous experiences. Extrinsic factors might include enforced changes to working patterns which you feel might have an adverse effect on your working life.

Finally

Having undertaken this exercise, discuss your findings with a colleague or fellow student nurse who knows you well, and whom you can trust to give you an honest and fair appraisal of how you have portrayed yourself. Once you are satisfied that your SWOT analysis is fair, you can begin to set out targets focusing on the legislative and policy initiatives that have been discussed. You can formulate a Personal Development Plan (PDP) which will enable you to respond to the policies and be equipped for changing practice delivery.

Box 3.3   Need to Know More?

Evans (2002) regards the Personal Development Plan (PDP) as a useful tool to enable nurses of all grades to gain the opportunity to pay attention to their career aspirations. PDPs are personal documents in which individuals can assess their current career. According to Evans, compiling a personal development plan can:

- Identify where you are now
- Encourage you to recognise your strengths and areas to improve
- Motivate you to set realistic and achievable goals
- Provide a tool to evaluate your achievements.

There are seven steps to drawing up a PDP. These are:

1   Review yourself
2   Plan to achieve
3   Draw up goals
4   Document your PDP
5   Identify resources to help you
6   Record your learning
7   Assess your achievements.

You will see that the work you have undertaken in your SWOT analysis will help you to formulate your PDP. It is essential that all of your actions are recorded in a portfolio, so that you can keep track of your achievements. This will provide reassurance that you are 'on track' with your achievements and remind you when you may have veered away from the targets set. The PDP will help you to achieve your goal of becoming better equipped for multi-professional working. You could consider the CNO's ten key roles for nurses, set out in Box 3.2 as a point of reference for the direction in which you might like your career to develop. It may also be useful to return to this exercise after completing this book to see if your developmental needs have changed.

Conclusion

This chapter has examined some of the most important legislation which has had an impact on multi-professional working in the primary care arena. It has also shown how traditional approaches to working have been challenged by innovative alliances, such as the collaborative working that takes place within the National Dementia Strategy and joint ventures with Boots the Chemist. It has also discussed changing relationships between medical and nursing professions in areas of Nurse Prescribing and Resuscitation. It has also given you the opportunity to consider how a community works and to undertake an exercise in Community Needs Assessment of the area in which you work. In addition, there was an explanation of SWOT analysis and an introduction to Personal Development Planning, both including activities designed to enable you to think about the ways in which you work now and how you intend to pursue your future career in nursing. The following chapters will offer further perspectives on the multi-professional nursing role and where and when this is likely to take place. Future services are likely to be radically different and, in order to be effective, getting to grips with new partnerships and service models is vital.

4

Multi-professional Working in the Community
Colin Goble

By reading this chapter you should be able to:

- **develop further what is meant by the term 'community'**
- **identify the main ideological and policy agendas shaping modern community-based health and social care**
- **identify the challenges and complexities of multi-professional working in the community**
- **identify the key knowledge and skills required to address and overcome these challenges and complexities**
- **identify how to work effectively in line with a person-centred ethos.**

Introduction

This chapter will focus on multi-professional practice in a community based context. Previous chapters have shown the need for a knowledge and understanding of other professions and agencies, and awareness and development of the skills for effective multi-professional working are regarded as vital for nursing in the modern health service context. The need for this knowledge and skill is nowhere greater than in a community based context, and the trend towards greater emphasis on community based health care provision means that this will become even more important in the future.

We will begin by defining what is meant by 'community', and by looking at the ways in which that term is used by differing ideological perspectives that have influenced the design and delivery of health and social care services. Then we will discuss how these ideas have been put into practice through the agendas of recent governments, focusing particularly on the modernisation agenda of New Labour, and the influence on that agenda of the 'social model of disability' and the move towards a 'primary care led' health service.

Some of the complexities and challenges involved in multi-professional working in the community will be explored: how these can be addressed and overcome by focusing work within a 'person-centred' ethos in which the interests of patients/clients are made paramount will be examined. This discussion will involve identifying the key knowledge base and skills involved in achieving what Beresford and Trevillion (1995) have described as 'a culture of collaboration'.

First then, there is a need to define and clarify what is meant by 'community'.

Defining a 'community'

At first glance, the meaning of the term 'community' might seem rather obvious and if you have read Chapter 3 you may have undertaken some work on this topic already. You will know that closer investigation reveals it to be a rather more complex and contentious concept, with important debates arising around questions such as 'What is the community?', 'Where is the community?', 'Who is the community?' and 'What does it mean to organise and provide health and social care in the community?' Beresford and Trevillion (1995) argue that the 'collectivist' model of welfare provision that underpinned the foundation of the Welfare State in the UK, and which remained dominant up until the 1970s, was based on the paternalistic idea that 'the community' was synonymous with 'the state' at both local and national level. According to this idea if a health or social care service was provided by 'the state' then this could be seen as 'the community' caring *for* its citizens. An image that can be associated with this idea, perhaps, is the idea of the community nurse travelling around a local patch, visiting and treating people in their home – until or if their condition became too serious then they would be moved into hospital. This model assumed that 'the hospital' was the main site for the delivery of serious and acute health care, and that health care in the 'community' was essentially about managing recuperation from hospital treatment, or monitoring chronic conditions.

However, the 'collectivist' model of service provision came under increasing attack from the 1960s onwards. Despite the cosy image alluded to above, the reality was that services could all too often be inefficient and oppressive in nature, with little regard given to the individual needs and desires of patients or services users. Beresford and Trevillion (1995) describe this as the 'isolated expert system', characterised by high levels of professional power, dominated by expert belief systems, indirect and 'reactive' communication between professionals, poor communication with service users and informal carers, and little professional accountability outside of formal management systems.

In 1979 the election of a Conservative government influenced by a 'New Right' political agenda saw a radical shift in the organisation of health and social care based on a very different conceptualisation of the 'community'. The traditional collectivist notion of the community as synonymous with the state was replaced by a 'neo-liberal' idea of the community as a loose-knit collection of competing individuals, usually living in families, and the associated belief that it was, therefore, families who should take primary responsibility for care and support of their vulnerable relatives. Where they could not do so, the private and voluntary sector, rather than the state, should be encouraged to provide services, particularly where what is required is long term care and support. This model was applied, in particular, to services for older people, people with learning disabilities and people with mental health problems, and has been described as care *in* the community, rather than care *by* the community (Baggott, 1988).

More recently there has been a further shift of emphasis, as the New Labour government elected in 1997 has pursued a policy agenda influenced by the so-called 'third way' political philosophy. This combines elements of both the 'collectivist' and 'neo-liberal' perspectives and sees the community as an expression of the collective responsibility of individuals and their families. From this perspective health and social care services are seen as part of the support mechanisms by which society both cares for vulnerable individuals and seeks to empower them as citizens. This model combines ideas both of care *for* and care *by*, the community, while also emphasising increasing levels of involvement and choice for patients/clients as empowered users of services. These have all become important elements in New Labour's 'modernisation' agenda.

Guided Study 4.1

From your reading so far think about the following questions:

- What do you understand by the term 'community' and why is this a contested term?
- What is the main difference between the 'collectivist' and 'neo-liberal' models of community, and why are these differences important for nurses to know about?
- What ideas have influenced the so called 'third way' approach to community based health care?

You could have included:

- Changing political ideas about the relationship between government, the state, and ordinary people who use health and social care services.
- How these ideas have been translated into policies and reforms affecting the way in which community based care is organised and delivered.
- The combination of the ideas of care *by* and care *in* the community.

Service user empowerment reflects the influence of another agenda affecting health and social care services that has emerged in recent decades from an increasingly politically active disability movement – an agenda based on the 'social model of disability'. We will now explore this agenda and the perspective on which it is based as a case study, first to grasp the significance of the challenge it presents to traditional nursing and health care practice, and, second, because of its impact on multi-professional working. As discussed below, recent policy initiatives suggest that this agenda is becoming a significant driving force behind the future organisation and provision of support for many client groups.

The challenge from the social model of disability

For much of the twentieth century the idea that disability was a purely bio-medical phenomenon, equivalent in most respects to disease, and therefore in need of similar programmes of eradication and treatment, went unquestioned. This kind of perspective tended to view the caring professions uncritically as part of a natural and rational response to social problems: a form of 'institutionalised altruism'. The growth of the independent living movement among physically disabled people in the 1970s and 1980s, however, led to a redefinition of disability first formally articulated in the UK by the Union of the Physically Impaired against Segregation (UPIAS, 1976). This definition replaced the term 'disability' with 'impairment' to describe the functional limitation experienced by an individual, while the use of the term 'disability' was altered to describe '… the limitations imposed on people with impairments by a society which fails to recognise, and/or organise itself to meet their needs'. Disability becomes, according to this definition, a category of social oppression similar to that associated with gender and race (Oliver, 1996).

The disability movement has used this type of analysis to organise politically to press for legislative change to defend and extend the rights of disabled people, including the right to have their views and perspectives listened to in health and social care services. This is a trend which is gaining influence at the highest political level. Recent policy developments promoting 'direct payments', where clients take control of their own service budget and buy the services they feel they need (DoH, 2003a), and the emphasis given to advocacy and inclusion in the *Valuing People* White Paper relating to people with learning disabilities (DoH, 2001d) are examples that illustrate that only those professions who open a dialogue, and demonstrate a genuine sense of solidarity, with disabled people are likely to survive and thrive in the future welfare state.

Guided Study 4.2

What is the impact of the 'social model of disability'?

You could have included:

- Changes in the balance of power between health and social care professionals including nurses and patients/clients.
- The way disabled people are challenging the traditional way that health and social care professionals have dealt with them, and the way they want this to change in the future – by, for example, having control over what kind of service they receive, who provides it, and where and when it is delivered.

The 'primary care' agenda

Another significant trend affecting the context of nursing and multi-professional practice in the community is that of the 'primary care led' model of health care provision. The 'primary care led' agenda emerged under the Conservative government in the early 1990s as part of a wider strategy concerned with shifting the emphasis of NHS provision away from expensive 'secondary care' based in hospitals, towards 'preventative care', where more health care functions – including diagnosis, assessment, surgery, post-operative care and long term management of chronic conditions – can be performed in local health centres and community based settings. Cost effectiveness and efficiency have been important arguments in the thinking behind this shift, but it has also fitted well with the World Health Organisation's (WHO) stated aim of shifting global health care provision away from a medicalised 'sickness' orientation, towards a holistic 'health promotion' model, with primary care services taking a lead role (WHO, 1978). In the UK, the *Health of the Nation: A Strategy for Health in England* White Paper (DoH, 1992a) represented the Government's response to this agenda, setting targets designed to meet the WHO's wider targets for health in Europe (WHO, 1985).

As Rick Fisher pointed out in the previous chapter, the trend towards a 'primary care led' NHS has continued and, indeed, been extended under 'New Labour', although with a shift of emphasis towards eradicating inequalities in health, and connected to a wider policy strategy to combat 'social exclusion' (DoH, 1997). Importantly for multi-professional working, there has also been a new emphasis on improving cooperation and collaboration between agencies, services and professionals (DoH, 1999b). Thus, the overall trend of government policy continues to be towards greater integration of health and social care services, with Health and Social Care Trusts being created to streamline management and administration, reduce conflict, and enhance collaborative working between professions (Wall and Owen, 2002).

For nurses, these reforms – and the service reorganisations that have accompanied them – have resulted in major changes, amounting in some cases to a complete redefinition of role, purpose and work setting. Learning disability nursing, for example, has been completely transformed from a profession based mainly in large institutions, performing a role that often amounted to little more than 'caring custody', to an almost entirely community based profession working across a wide range of services – residential, respite, primary care, educational – in a wide range of health and social care orientated roles, and for a wide range of service providers – not just the NHS (Gates, 2003). Many other nurses in adult, children's and mental health services are also experiencing significant changes and the drive towards a 'primary care led' NHS and integrated services is likely to mean that these trends will continue, to the extent that for nurses 'working in the community' may well become the norm, rather than the exception.

Guided Study 4.3

What is the likely impact of a 'primary care led' context of care on nurses and their partnerships within the community?

You could have included:

- Nursing of all kinds is likely to become increasingly community, rather than hospital based in the future.

(Continued)

(Continued)

- Nurses are increasingly likely to work in, or have involvement with, a greater variety of service providers – not just the NHS – than previously.
- Nurses will increasingly work in integrated services, with a breakdown of the organisational and professional barriers between 'health' and 'social' care, and other services too, such as education.
- Nursing will involve increasing levels of multi-professional and inter-agency contact and working.
- Patient/client influence and control over services will increase significantly, with major implications for nursing roles and practice.

Having looked at how nursing in the community has changed, and will continue to do so, let us now focus on multi-professional working itself.

Challenges for multi-professional working – a person centred approach

In Chapter 1 the reform and reorganisation of the community care context in which professional health and social care work was noted. You have seen that a shift away from large institutional, state run, models of care for groups of people with long term care and support needs to smaller scale services dispersed in the community, or based in the patient/client's family home has changed the focus of service delivery. This has been particularly true of services for people with learning disabilities, older people, people with mental health problems and people with physical and sensory impairments. An important component of this shift away from institutional models of care has been a move towards a 'person centred' model of support (Gates, 2006).

Person centred approaches to care and support have received significant government backing in policy directed towards community care, such as the *Valuing People* White paper for people with learning disabilities (DoH, 2001d). More recently, *High Quality Care For All* (DOH, 2008b) embraces further the need for all services to be personalised (DOH, 2008b: 18). Effective multi-professional working is a vital component in making person centred approaches work, requiring collaboration between a variety of professions and agencies. Managing relationships between these professions and agencies can be complex. Some major challenges for multi-professional working include, for example:

- *Managing power relationships* – For instance, with doctors and service managers (who may well also be a health professional, such as a nurse). Both these groups have, and need, to exercise power and authority in order to fulfil their roles, but the priorities of both may differ, with doctors prioritising clinical and treatment issues, while managers prioritise operational, organisational and financial issues.

- *Differing and potentially competing roles between organisations and professions in the health and social care 'market'* – One of the effects of the new types of partnership in community care has been to create the potential for conflict and competition between professions over certain areas of work with various patient and client groups – for example, competition between social workers and nurses over who assesses the needs of people with mental health problems. A relatively new phenomenon is the emergence of a new breed of health and social care worker who has risen through the ranks outside the traditional forms of professional training, with qualifications based on vocational, work-based training, such as national vocational qualifications (NVQs), rather than traditional professional routes of training, a trend increasingly endorsed and promoted by government policy over the past decade (for instance, DoH, 1999b: TOPSS, 2000).

- *Variation in the traditions and cultures of various service agencies* – The NHS, social services, and the so-called 'third' and private sector organisations all have different histories, cultures and priorities that mean that their ways of working also differ, sometimes considerably. Many 'third sector' organisations, for example, have their origins in voluntary and charity organisations which have traditionally been strongly influenced by parents and carers of particular client groups. This means that they have high levels of commitment towards their client groups, but perhaps lack a tradition of professional organisation and management; indeed, they may have an almost 'anti-professional' ethos based on years of fighting official systems on behalf of their patient/client group. This sector is becoming increasingly important, however, particularly in social care, and the trend of managerialisation that began in state sector health and social care in the 1980s is now reaching into this sector as part of the extension of the government's modernisation agenda for public services (Hudson, 2002). For nurses, whether working for, or in interaction with, organisations in this sector, the priority is to be aware of, and sensitive to, their varying histories, cultures and traditions, and the impact this may have on their way of working. In Chapter 9 Terry Scragg will explore this emerging sector in more detail.

- *The varying cultures, histories and philosophies of different professions* – As introduced in Chapter 1, different professions have differing cultures, histories and philosophies. For example doctors often work from a problem solving orientation, emphasising technical, treatment based approaches and outcomes, whereas social work has a more social science-oriented knowledge base, emphasising skills such as interpersonal communication, and concepts such as 'anti-oppressive practice'. At least part of the historical orientation of social work has been 'anti-medical' as well, particularly in relation to groups such as people with learning disabilities with whom the orientation of care and support has shifted under community care reforms from a 'medical' to 'social' model. Some branches of nursing – such as learning disability nursing – have found themselves straddling this 'health and social' care divide, struggling at times to identify their role and identity (Turnball, 2004).

- *Many professionals are defensive and cynical after years of change and sometimes outright attack* – A feature of the politics of health and social care in the latter half of the twentieth century, continuing into the first decade of the twenty-first century, has been critiques of the caring professions that have come from both the political 'left' and 'right'. The left have tended to criticise the caring professions from the perspective of solidarity with 'service users'; an example being the 'disability movement' who have argued, as you saw above, for a redefinition of disability as a form of oppression rather than as a form of bio-medical diagnosis. This means thinking about how, historically, professional behaviour and service systems have sometimes oppressed and disempowered people by taking control over their lives, such as making people with learning disabilities live in large, isolated institutions, separated from wider society, denying them access to education, work, or even the opportunity to get married, for example (French and Swain, 2001). Alternatively, critiques from 'the right' have emphasised the way in which professions can become entrenched self-interest groups which gain control over resources and systems in health and social care, producing inefficient and wasteful forms of practice, and disempowering service users by restricting choice. It is this critique which, as you saw earlier, lay behind the market orientated model of community care that has emerged in the UK, though the 'left' critique has also been influential at a cultural and philosophical level. One result of these critiques, however, is that many in the caring and nursing professions in community services have tended to develop a 'siege' mentality, leading to cynicism and a tendency at times to be resistant to change (Baggot, 1988).

Guided Study 4.4

Think about your practice experience in a community based setting. Do you recognise any of the challenges identified above in what you saw? In particular, think about the interaction of different professionals and service agencies. Were there any 'tensions', and if so why do you think this was? Were these tensions addressed or ignored and what was the impact of this?

You could have included:

- The way in which the professionals you observed talked about each other, and/or the organisations they work for – both 'officially' and 'unofficially' – and what this told you about how they see other professions and/or organisations.
- The way the professionals you observed exercised power in their interactions – constructively or otherwise – and the effect this had on the way the team worked.
- The way in which the interaction of the professionals and organisations you observed could be made to work more smoothly and effectively.

This last point should get you thinking about how to overcome problems and challenges in multi-professional working; an area you will now focus on.

Overcoming the challenges

Many of the challenges raised above may seem complex and negative; however, the person centred approach offers one of the best ways to work through these challenges by placing the patient/client at the centre of professional thinking and systems. Person centred practice requires a particular commitment in nurses and other health and social care professionals to operationalise. For example, a strong set of shared values and professional attitudes that value service users as 'the experts' on their own situation is required, underpinned by relevant and evidence based knowledge which needs to be translated into specific skills. We will now look at each of these areas – values, attitudes, knowledge and skills – in turn, and how they can enhance your multi-professional working in community based health and social care services.

Values for multi-professional working in the community

It has been argued that in an organisational and political climate of almost constant change, it is 'values' that provide consistency and continuity (Brown and Cambridge, 1995). Underpinning the shift to community care has been a moral/philosophical commitment to caring for and supporting vulnerable people in home-like environments – preferably in their own home – and in an individualised, 'person centred' manner that encourages maximum independence and autonomy. The term 'autonomy' is key here, as it emphasises that independence for service users should be about much more than just the ability to maintain self-care – such as washing and feeding the self – but should also be about choice, and control in decision making – even if this sometimes conflicts with professional views and judgements. It is this commitment to the pursuit of autonomous control for the service user, or the nearest thing to it – via systems of family, citizen or independent advocacy for example – that is at the heart of 'person-centred' approaches to care and support, and it is this commitment that needs to be the agreed cornerstone for multi-professional groups and teams working to support individuals in community settings. Beresford and Trevillion (1995) point out that collaborative working is most effective among professionals when they work from a shared value base, and communicating and establishing this value base can therefore be seen as the foundation of effective multi-professional practice.

Professional attitudes towards multi-professional working

Up to now this chapter has presented what might be seen as a rather 'anti-professional' perspective. It is important to remember, however, that health and social care professionals have often been at the forefront of promoting service users' rights and improvements to services. The term 'professionalism' has multiple meanings, and although professions are often looked at critically, they can and should also be viewed positively. For example, professionalism can be seen as a benchmark of performance, competence and moral quality. Friedson (1994) has argued that professions are, despite all the critiques, better than the alternatives and are both necessary and desirable to maintain a 'decent' society.

It can be argued then that it is not 'professionalism' in itself that is the problem, but the attitude with which professionals approach their role in people's lives. One way to develop a new, empowering kind of professionalism, which attempts to address and overcome the shortcomings of traditional, paternalistic forms of professionalism is by adopting an attitude of solidarity with, rather than control over, patients and clients. This requires a 'dialogue' based approach to the development of professional knowledge and practice, drawing in particular from the experience of individual patients and clients, and their representative groups; a view that echoes the perspectives of the social model of disability. Such an approach needs to be continuously promoted in those forums and systems where health and social care professionals interact, thus ensuring that an empowering attitude is carried into the multi-disciplinary working context. In this way professional attitudes can be aligned to ensure that they become part of the solution, rather than a continuing part of the problem.

Relevant knowledge and awareness for multi-professional working in the community

Carnaby and Cambridge (2006) have argued that a sound knowledge base for staff is one of the keys to ensuring quality in community based services. Thompson and Mathias (1998) identified a number of crucial areas of knowledge and awareness that need to be developed by health and social professionals working in multi-professional contexts in the community. These include knowledge and awareness of the following issues.

Current social and service policy

Knowledge and awareness of the policy context is important for all health and social care professionals so that they understand the context within which they work. Ideally, it should also form the basis of an involvement in helping to shape that context for the future. Such knowledge and awareness is important in developing an empowered practice, influencing how services function, and how professional roles can be shaped in line with patient and client needs and priorities. As you have seen, the emphasis on multi-professional and collaborative working is itself policy driven, and has emerged because of problems in this area of professional and service operation in the past – problems that have often left patients/clients and their carers without an adequate service or support. If nurses and other professionals are to be part of the solution, rather than perpetuating the problem, then a commitment from them to making it work effectively is necessary.

Roles of other professionals

To work effectively with other professionals on behalf of patients and clients in the community, a knowledge and awareness of, and respect for, what other professions do, and how their knowledge and skills can be used, is vital. Opportunities to develop this knowledge and awareness are an important element of learning experiences for student health and social care professionals, and there is a welcome trend towards collaborative and joint learning in professional training. If you have read Chapter 2 you may have participated in the guided study activity around professional roles in services for older people. Sometimes, however, there may be the potential for conflict between professions which may sour this relationship. The solution to such tensions may not be easy to resolve, but neither should they be used to fuel conflicts in ways that use patients/clients as political pawns in professional power struggles. Where such conflicts exist, a 'person-centred' commitment requires professionals to avoid situations where patients/clients are involved, and use other channels of multi-professional dialogue and negotiation to resolve them.

Procedures, structures and systems

A knowledge and awareness of service procedures, structures and systems is important for nurses for a variety of reasons. For example, linked to the knowledge and awareness of the roles of other professionals discussed above, this knowledge can be extremely useful in helping patients/clients gain access to the services of other professionals who can help them with particular aspects of the care and support they require. It may also help the nurse in being able to advocate on behalf of their patient/client to gain such support where this is not happening. Such knowledge is also important if nurses are to contribute to the further development of procedures, structures and systems which enhance the quality of service provision and collaboration for the benefit of patients and clients. For instance, Carnaby and Cambridge (2006) point out the importance of information sharing and communication between professionals and carers, both 'formal' and 'informal', in ensuring that the needs of people with severe learning difficulties and communication difficulties are met. This can be as basic as ensuring an accurate handover of information between residential and day services about what a person has eaten in order to maintain satisfactory nutrition, or as complex as conducting a holistic assessment that captures information from a variety of professional perspectives; but to achieve either requires the establishment of clear lines, modes and records of communication that ensures both quality and accountability. Procedures, structures and systems should thus be designed to enhance, rather than inhibit, multi-professional collaboration, and where they don't, a knowledge of how this can be changed and used to achieve better outcomes is an important component of the leadership and managerial aspects of nursing knowledge and roles.

Guided Study 4.5

Think about your experience of multi-professional working in community based settings. Think about the service procedures you saw in action. How effective were they? Did they work well or were there problems? If so, why do you think this was? How important do you think communication between professionals and services were in making things work well?

(Continued)

(Continued)

You could have included:

- The importance of knowing about the roles of other professionals and agencies.
- How to access and communicate with other professionals and agencies on a regular basis.
- The importance of meeting other professionals regularly to develop friendly and cooperative relationships.
- The importance of focusing on meeting the needs of patients and clients above all else.

Funding and budgeting controls and constraints

A knowledge of financial issues and systems is increasingly important for a number of reasons. For example, community care in the UK is primarily organised around financial management systems. The system of 'Care Management' established by the NHS and Community Act (1990) was designed as a mechanism to both control and target spending towards patients/clients on the basis of assessed need. Thus, assessment of patient/client need has become firmly linked to budget allocation and, to put it at its most simple – it is only possible within this system to purchase services that have actually been assessed against care or support needs. Given that professional nursing care is among the more costly of services that can be allocated under this system it is important that any care provided is cost effective. For nurses this means that they need to be aware of the cost implications of their own interventions and of their interactions with other professionals and agencies. The advent and increasing use of 'direct payments', where service users take greater control of their own budgets and buy the services they feel they need, looks set to change the landscape still further, and will no doubt concentrate the minds of all in the caring professions about how they can demonstrate their cost effectiveness to their patient/client employers.

Multi-professional and inter-organisational communication

Communication is central to the whole process of person centred care and support, and linked to the most important skills in multi-professional working. Recent decades have seen a major revolution in communication technologies in the industrialised world that should work to facilitate multi-professional communication in health and social care. The government has invested hugely in information and communication technologies in the NHS and across the public services. The results have not always been as spectacular or successful as promised, and there are many issues relating to the design and compatibility of IT and communication systems. What is not in doubt, however, is that knowledge of how to use these technologies is no longer optional, but essential for nurses and other health and social care professionals. The introduction of technology has not altered the essentials of good and effective communication, however, and the best results are still achieved by the well-established virtues of talking to people, building trust and establishing reliability and accessibility. It is here that knowledge of, and respect for, other professions and agencies, their procedures, structures and systems – including those related to finance – comes into its own.

Group and team dynamics, leadership styles, and decision making processes

Multi-professional care and support is usually organised in groups and teams, which can be complex. Knowledge and awareness of how groups and teams work is necessary in order to ensure that they do so effectively. It is here that power relationships between professions can become influential, and need careful management. For instance, as explored in Chapter 1, senior doctors can often assume the leadership and control of multi-professional groups and teams by default and based on a number of assumptions about professional hierarchies. Sometimes this may be for the best, but not necessarily, and the balancing presence and leadership of other senior professionals or managers can be useful to make a group or team work more effectively, particularly in a community care setting where medical priorities may not be the most important. The chairing, leadership and management of groups and teams is an important part of the skills required by senior nurses working in the community and, once again, a 'person-centred' emphasis, with patient/client need made a priority, should work to ensure that a group or team keeps its focus and maximises its effectiveness. Chapters 7 and 10 will help you build your knowledge of leading teams and work with any conflict that may be present.

Your own role and position in systems and team

While knowledge and skills in leadership and management of groups and teams, and their decision making processes is important for senior nurses, all nurses need to develop a sound awareness and knowledge of their own place within the service and in teams. This will help you to operate with confidence to gain the trust and respect of other professionals and agencies – essential ingredients of effective multi-professional working.

Working in anti-oppressive and anti-discriminatory ways

Nursing has only comparatively recently taken on board the necessity for focusing on anti-oppressive and anti-discriminatory working as part of its training, and some other professions – notably social work – have traditionally given much greater emphasis to developing these areas of professional knowledge and practice. An essential element of 'person centred' working is the necessity of identifying actual and potentially oppressive and discriminatory ideas and perceptions which may influence our actions and behaviours towards patients and clients – an issue of particular importance given the cultural, gender/sexuality and ability/disability diversity, both of patients and clients, and of other professionals and carers. Anti-oppressive and anti-discriminatory practice is not something that can be 'learned' and ticked off, however, but requires a constant and periodic individual and collective reflection on the ways people work and interact – a practice that should itself be built into the multi-professional group and team working.

How to work with and manage change

Constant and ongoing organisational change has become a part of the reality within which nursing operates in modern community based health and social care systems. The shift to a community based emphasis in health and social care is itself a reflection of this, as is the increasing and still developing role of private and 'third sector' organisations. The service-user led agenda now being given emphasis will undoubtedly lead to further change in the shape and organisation of services and professional roles. Dealing with constant change can be stressful and, if not well managed, lead to demoralisation and cynicism. One of the best antidotes to this is to remain focused on the strong values underpinning person centred approaches to working. Nursing is, after all, about promoting positive change in the lives and well-being of patients/clients. Maintaining this focus should help you to deal with your own response to the ongoing change you experience.

Relevant research and evidence based practice

The move towards an 'evidence based practice' culture in nursing, and in the health and social care field generally, has been another feature of the broad government-driven modernisation agenda in recent years. Two main interlinked factors that underlie it are: the drive for cost effectiveness – by focusing resources on what is known to work and produce the most effective outcomes; and the 'professionalisation' agenda in nursing and other health and social care professions – where the focus is on demonstrating to the 'powers that be' that the profession has a scientifically validated knowledge base, and is thus worth investing in to meet the need of patients/clients. A third, perhaps more significant factor for many nurses, is the desire to do what works best for patients/clients. Evidence based practice covers a wide range of techniques and practices, including those relating to effective multi-professional working, and it is to those practices – or skills – that we turn.

Skills for multi-professional working in the community

It is perhaps stating the obvious that the skills involved in multi-professional working are primarily those of managing effective and respectful working relationships. Many of the skills involved are the same whatever the working context. Working in the community adds some extra factors, making practice more complex. The main issues, as have been discussed, relate to working across differing organisational and professional cultures, and across settings that are often geographically dispersed. A 'person centred' ethos requires that nurses therefore work consciously to avoid tendencies towards professional 'tribalism', and avoid slipping into the 'isolated expert' system of working identified by Beresford and Trevillion (1995) and referred to earlier. Those authors undertook an extensive study in which users of community care services identified those skills in professions which they most valued. These are outlined below as part of the essential building blocks of what Beresford and Trevillion describe as a 'collaborative culture' for practice.

Towards a collaborative culture

Building a collaborative culture in the community requires a focus on the communication skills which will help to develop trust and good relationships with other professionals, organisations, patients/clients themselves and their families and relatives. Such skills are integral to the person centred approach, needed to adopt in providing care and support for patients/client living in the community. Among the most important of these skills are:

- **Assertiveness skills** – The ability to be able to assert your own point of view or perspective in a way that is perceived by others as confident, rather than arrogant and/or aggressive. The key to a good assertive style of working involves developing a good level of self-awareness, focusing on awareness of body posture, use of appropriate language and the ability to actively listen and assimilate the views and perspectives of others. It also involves knowing your limits – being confident enough to say 'I don't know', avoiding the use of jargon and technical/professional language wherever possible, using an explanatory communication style and staying focused on finding solutions.
- **Advocacy skills** – Advocacy is part of the nursing role, but it is one that needs to be approached with some caution. It is particularly important to recognise the potential conflicts between the role of 'advocate' and the role of 'professional'. A professional nurse is also, inevitably, a representative of the organisation they work for and the nursing profession itself. These are 'interests' that can potentially conflict with the needs and desires of the patient/client. The first stage of planning an advocacy intervention therefore is to ask the question 'Am I the right person to do the advocating?' A 'person centred' focus may require us to accept that our patient/client's interests are better served by an advocate who is independent of organisational and professional interests that may constrain us. As a rule, professional advocacy is probably best restricted to 'service level' advocacy – that is advocating for access to the skills/expertise of other professionals within or across

different services. It is here that the knowledge about other professional roles, systems of referral, finance and of one's own position within an organisational context referred to above will come into its own. This, combined with an informed and up to date knowledge of treatments, interventions and services which may help your patient/client to meet their assessed needs, will form the basis of your 'case'. Key skills will be those involved in the preparation and presentation of this case to the appropriate forum.

- **Negotiation skills** – The complexities of multi-professional working, whatever the context, tend to revolve around negotiating who will do what, how, by when and who will pay for it. A crucial aspect of doing this effectively involves the ability to recognise potential points of conflict, heading them off wherever possible and resolving them effectively where conflict does arise. In particular, it is vital to avoid entering into a negotiation with the idea that one party will 'win' and the other will 'lose'. Instead, a problem-solving approach needs to be adopted from the start, with the aim of everyone focused on meeting the needs of the patient/client in the most satisfactory way possible. The skills relating to both assertiveness and advocacy referred to above may come into play here, but negotiation processes will be made a great deal easier if there exists a good level of trust and mutual respect. Thus, establishing good lines of communication outside of the negotiation context, and time spent building good rapport – visiting and introducing oneself, outlining your own role and perspective, and establishing a 'common cause' by emphasising your commitment to a person centred approach – will be well spent.

- **Acting and working in a business-like manner** – All of the above will be greatly helped if your own approach to your work is grounded in behaviours associated with 'professionalism'. Behaviours which demonstrate reliability, punctuality and willing participation in operational processes of delegation and workload division will all contribute to demonstrating your commitment to making collaboration work.

- **Encouraging information sharing** – Another aspect of a business-like approach to multi-professional working is information sharing. Control of information and its dissemination is one of the ways in which professions have traditionally engaged in practices of 'isolationism' and 'tribalism'. The development of a collaborative culture requires a commitment to behavioural change – chief among which is the way that information is stored, shared and disseminated. The aim should be that the correct information is shared at the right time and in the right format among the people who need to know in order to achieve the best outcomes for the patient/client. The need to protect sensitive information in line with legal and ethical requirements is also paramount. Key skills in this area will involve verbal, written and electronic presentation, together with the use of computer and information technology.

- **Constructive advice, supervision and mentoring** – Good support and governance systems are an essential component in making multi-professional work successful. The skills of advising, supervising and mentoring staff and other team members, sometimes from other professions and other organisations are, therefore, an increasingly important part of the skills of the professional nurse. It is also important, however, to ensure that you receive good supervisory and mentoring support – particularly if you are to remain reflective about your own practice. Joint and collaborative forums for multi-professional discussion and reflection are a particularly useful way of sharing information and knowledge about each other's professional perspectives, skills and practice, and an opportunity to develop a sense of shared commitment to person centred methods and approaches to meeting patient/client needs.

- **Involvement of patient/client in person centred approaches to working** – Beresford and Trevillion (1995) placed commitment to the involvement of patients/clients at the centre of their strategy for creating a collaborative culture and practice. In their research, they identified a number of key components to achieving this, including allowing the space and time for such involvement, dependent on whatever level the patient/client is able or willing to be involved; a commitment to including the patient/client, or their advocate or representative in decision making, at *all* levels, including, and especially, those around important life choices; avoidance of the use of professional jargon, and keeping technical language to its appropriate context; and a commitment to not sacrifice individual or collective patient/client interests in multi-professional power play, point scoring or disputes, but rather to be led by the needs of the patient/client. Cally Ward takes this further in Chapter 6.

The skills outlined here are those that nurses need to develop, alongside their clinical knowledge and expertise, to ensure that they operate effectively in the community based, multi-professional context that is the shape of the increasingly integrated health and social care services to come. They should also form the basis for a new type of professionalism, based on a commitment to working collaboratively with patients and clients to identify and meet their needs on an individualised and personalised basis.

Conclusion

In this chapter you have looked at multi-professional working in the community. You have seen that the nature and policy context of nursing in the community has changed radically over recent decades, and the drive towards a greater emphasis on community based multi-professional working is continuing within a policy agenda of increased collaboration and integration of health and social care services. A number of challenges and changes have been highlighted. By focusing on the knowledge, values and skills required to work effectively in these new contexts, and by placing the patient/client at the centre of your approach to multi-professional work, you can ensure that your practice does not lose sight of its central purpose despite the complexity of the community context.

5

Nursing and Multi-professional Practice in the Acute Sector
Sid Carter

By reading this chapter you should be able to:

- **identify legislation and practices that impact on the nurse's role in multi-professional working in acute care**
- **explore the tensions and complexities of team working in acute care**
- **reflect on your own multi-professional values as you participate in guided study activity from social psychology**
- **extend your knowledge of communication strategies by exploring evidence-based examples from practice**
- **access websites to learn more about nursing and models of multi-professional working in the acute sector.**

Introduction

This chapter examines the place of multi-professional working in acute health care against the backdrop of real life complexities. The drive for professionals to work more cooperatively in a number of health care settings – including benefits and difficulties – have been explored. Here, processes that can make or break efforts to create teamwork in acute care will be examined, and you will be invited to participate in a number of guided study activities to explore this from your perspective.

Very human factors of pride, prejudice, fear of ridicule and a desire to belong to a group can be vital in working relationships just as much as in everyday life. A consistent theme throughout is the centrality of good communication. The needs of patients in acute care can change very rapidly, and have the added complexity of potentially involving a large number of people, especially at the interface with discharging patients into social care. Each one of these people needs to keep in touch with the fast changing picture of a patient's needs, and you will see that this demanding level of communication relies on the flexibility and mutual trust of the individuals involved.

Professional roles in acute care have changed in recent years. There are new types of professional, for example the Emergency Care Practitioner (ECP), and established professions are developing in different directions. For example, the work done by nurses has extended immensely, including nurse prescribing. New types of nursing roles have also emerged, such as the Advanced Nurse Practitioner (ANP). Griffin and Melby (2006) studied the attitudes of various professional groups towards the ANP role in Ireland, finding largely positive acceptance, with the exception of General Practitioners. Other extended nurse roles include Nurse Consultants (Woodward et al., 2006) and Modern Matrons (Savage and Scott 2004; Dealey et al., 2007).

Leathard (2003) recounts the fast and relentless programme of change through social policy and legislation to encourage collaboration at all levels of health and social care services. This pressure ranges from attempts to integrate health and social care at national level, through to encouraging professional collaboration at ward level. An example illustrating the depth of this desire for collaborative working is the growth of multi-professional education. The educational preparation of acute care professions was at one time very separate, but a growing number of programmes now contain large elements of shared learning. The effectiveness of multi-professional education programmes are currently being evaluated (Stone, 2006).

However, not all policy measures that endorse multi-professional working in the acute sector make it easy, as sometimes the aims of different policies are in conflict with each other. Miller and Freeman's (2003) research on multi-professional teams in acute settings found such a conflict between imperatives to keep bed occupancy high, and clinical governance objectives to improve communication between professional groups. Ensuring high bed occupancy meant patients from different specialities could be placed in several wards, meaning that professionals spent a lot of time moving from place to place to see them. This disrupted team relationships and gave less time for quality communication.

Examples of multi-professional working in acute health care practice

This section explores some examples from acute health care practice, demonstrating how vital multi-professional working is, and how it is often nurses who play a pivotal role in making it successful.

Nurse-facilitated discharge/single assessment discharge planning

Recent advances in discharge planning place nurses in a lead role in coordinating the efforts of other professionals. Single assessment discharge planning (DOH, 2002e) aimed to achieve more flexible working among different professional groups, to enable a more effective conclusion to each patient's care. This meant nurses working outside their expected boundaries, with both health and social care professionals.

Good quality discharge planning is a multi-professional activity, frequently led by nurses (Lees, 2007). The leadership element places a large responsibility on nurses, requiring a great deal of self-motivation. Lees (2004) suggested that the term 'nurse facilitated discharge' is preferable to 'nurse led discharge' as it is less likely to cause friction among other professionals. Whichever term is chosen, though, nurses responsible for discharge planning need a thorough knowledge of intermediate care, social care services and the contributions made by other disciplines. Without this knowledge and awareness, patients could find themselves wasting valuable time and resources in unsuitable services. You will have spent time learning about the roles of other professionals in earlier chapters.

The number of acute care beds in the NHS has reduced dramatically over the last two decades (Pollock and Dunnigan, 2000). Bed reduction means that discharge has to be quicker and more efficient, as new patients wait for their much-needed admissions, and the Department of Health has made the importance of this process very clear (Lees, 2006). Around 80 per cent of discharges are known as simple discharges, characterised by the successful treatment of a specific condition, followed by straightforward care when a patient returns home (DoH, 2004d). The remaining 20 per cent are complex discharges, featuring a complicated and ongoing medical status combined with complex care arrangements once the person has left hospital (Dyer and Temple, 2007).

Dyer and Temple (2007) present several factors that are crucial to the success of complex discharges. It is important to have clear leadership of the discharge process; this is likely to be best delegated to a nurse or therapist. Genuinely multi-professional ward rounds are crucial, including perhaps the most important factor overall: good communication.

Wade (2007) also emphasises the importance of communication among different professional groups in effective discharge planning. This naturally includes communicating with the patient and their family or carers, to make sure their views become part of the information available. Nurses can be well placed to facilitate this promotion of the patient's perspective, through good face-to-face communication and good record keeping.

In conclusion, because of limited hospital beds, effective acute care services depend on timely discharges. This means patients spending no more time in hospital than they have to. Fast, safe discharges in turn rely utterly on good multi-professional working.

Integrated care pathways

Integrated care pathways have become an important part of the delivery of acute health care, and usually involve a significant element of multi-professional collaboration. Integrated care pathways are also known by other names, for example, 'collaborative plan of care' and 'multi-disciplinary action plans', (for explanation of these definitions, see Chapter 1), but all have essentially the same structure. The key aim of an integrated care pathway is to produce a blueprint of the best possible care for a particular condition from beginning to end.

The European Pathway Association (EPA) has defined the critical elements of a clinical or care pathway, gaining international consensus (EPA, 2005, cited in Whittle 2006) as:

- Care pathways provide a method for the various groups of professionals involved to share the organisation of care, and decision making
- Pathways collate the best treatments for a particular condition, founded on the highest quality evidence and practice available
- Care pathways facilitate communication and collaboration between members of the multi-professional team
- Documentation is shared
- Resources are identified.

De Bleser et al. (2006) conducted an in-depth analysis of what professionals mean by the term 'care pathway', arriving at a framework similar to the EPA. De Bleser et al.'s analysis gave a clearer understanding of the ideas behind integrated care pathways. Top of the list was the idea of 'homogeneous patient group', not surprising since the intention is to create a best practice protocol for a specific condition. Coming a close second was the concept of 'multidisciplinary team', thus multi-professional working is at the heart of the care pathway approach to acute health care.

Olsson, et al. (2007) present an example of an integrated care pathway in action, demonstrating how the contributions of different professions can be orchestrated for the benefit of the patient. Olsson and colleagues compared the outcomes for two groups of older people with hip fractures. One group received standard care, and the other group's care was managed through a care pathway.

The hip fracture integrated care pathway included evidence based steps, with indicators of individuals falling behind their expected progress closely monitored by the multi-professional team, but particularly by nurses. An example of one of the steps in the integrated care pathway was the non-use or very early removal of catheters. This meant patients had to mobilise to use the bathroom, thus assisting their recovery.

Olsson et al.'s (2007) first measure to compare the success of the integrated care pathway group with the success of the standard care group was to return to pre-fracture levels of independence. This was based on very thorough questioning of patients on their self care abilities before their hip fracture. The integrated care pathway group achieved 21 per cent full restoration of activities of daily living, while the standard care group achieved 5 per cent. Olsson et al. suggested that integrated care pathways operate by constantly reminding professionals of the evidence based elements of the pathway, and the importance of each multi-professional contribution.

Atwal and Caldwell (2002) also studied the use of integrated care pathways in the treatment of hip fracture, finding that, overall, the care pathway approach benefited patients. However, they also discovered that there were various negative multi-professional processes that hampered the aims of the care pathway. These included reduced face-to-face communication, partly as a result of fear of the consequences of opposing colleagues. Another negative factor was the reduced participation in pathway activities by some professionals as they felt their 'professional identity' was threatened. Evaluations of integrated care pathway effectiveness are largely positive, but it may be factors that disrupt multi-professional working such as those discovered by Atwal and Caldwell that lead to their mixed success.

An example of the qualified success of integrated care pathways is provided by Kent and Chalmers (2006), who reviewed over 100 integrated care pathways implemented over a period of ten years in Scotland. Though largely successful, Kent and Chalmers attributed some of the failures to a lack of multi-professional motivation and the need for an individual locally to 'drive' the care pathway. This picture of mixed success can be found in other areas, demonstrated by a study of a diabetes care pathway in Scotland (Waller et al., 2007), and also hepatitis C (Fahey, 2007), and acute stroke care (Sulch and Kalra, 2000; Kwan et al., 2004).

Thus, although integrated care pathways bring together the best evidence based practices to specific areas of care, they still need good multi-professional working to achieve their full potential.

Venous thromboembolism: treatment and prevention

A venous thromboembolism (VTE, or more simply, a blood clot) can cause a blockage in the deep veins of the body's extremities, particularly the legs, causing deep vein thrombosis (DVT). This painful condition can lead to consequences that are more serious. Sometimes part of a clot in a leg vein breaks off, eventually blocking blood supply to the lungs, known as a pulmonary embolism (PE), which can be fatal. Around 25,000 people in England die each year from VTE following hospital admission, and VTE kills five times more people than hospital acquired infections (Sadler, 2007).

Current approaches to VTE benefit patients through a combination of biomedical advances in drug treatment with more creative multi-professional working. Cunnington (2003) described how VTE treatment has changed in recent years. At one time, patients who were thought to have a DVT were admitted to an acute hospital bed to have intravenous heparin while waiting for imaging. Imaging is the only sure way of diagnosing a DVT, as there are many possible causes for a swollen leg, for example, cellulitis (Carter et al., 2007b). Even if it was discovered that a patient did not have a DVT, they would have spent several days in hospital receiving an unnecessary treatment which in itself posed some health risks.

This unsatisfactory situation continued until the development of low molecular weight heparin (LMWH), which only requires a single subcutaneous injection per day. This enabled a change in service delivery, for example, a study by Rose et al. (2001) demonstrated that treatment for DVT could be delivered on an outpatient basis. Rose et al.'s multi-centre study used eight hospitals across the UK to trial LMWH, based in some of the developing outpatient DVT services, many of which were nurse-led.

Cunnington (2003) relates how DVT treatment with the advent of LMWH was mixed, using both inpatient and outpatient models. In her area (Leicester), a senior nurse led the establishment of an outpatient DVT service run by a specialist DVT nurse.

The specialist DVT nurse coordinated the input of various professionals, such as hospital doctors, radiographers and pharmacists. It was also necessary to enlist the cooperation of primary care health professionals, especially to encourage GPs to refer suspected DVT cases to the specialist service. Cunnington (2003) quantified the benefits to Leicester patients of the nurse-led multi-professional DVT service. In one year approximately 1,000 hospital bed days had been saved. Similar DVT services are now more widespread, for accounts see Davis (2005) (Wirral), and Sadler (2007) (Portsmouth).

Despite these advances in the treatment of VTE, it is still very prevalent and part of the strategy for dealing with it is prevention. NICE (2007a) issued guidelines on the prevention of VTE following surgery, with more general prevention guidelines being developed. Carter (2007) stated how VTE prevention is variable across services, and how assessment, appropriate protection and public awareness will help to make practice more consistent. More consistent VTE prevention requires good multi-professional practice to uphold standards.

Developments in the approach to the prevention and treatment of VTE are a good example of the importance of placing the service user at the centre of acute care. How individual patients actually feel about their care can so easily be left behind in the complex and high pressure environment of acute services. David Farrell was the patient representative on the group that developed NICE guidelines for the reduction of blood clots in surgical patients. When the guidelines were published, he said, 'Had this guideline been available when I underwent surgery on my knee, I may not have developed the blood clot that resulted in an unnecessary stint in hospital and took six months to recover from' (NICE, 2007b). This sort of example shows the importance of including the views of service users at a national level, but it is also vital at a local level. A lot of the material in this chapter concerns the difficulties of encouraging professionals to talk and listen to each other, which implies that listening properly to patients can also be difficult in an acute setting.

Guided Study 5.1

Think about your experiences in acute care settings. Have you noticed professionals going out of their way to take patients' views into account? What factors have you observed that make listening to patients more likely?

Is the patient more likely to be listened to when the different professions are working together collaboratively?

Working with partners

Teamwork

For you to understand how to work effectively in a multi-professional acute care setting, it is important to have some knowledge of how teams operate. A well-known model for analysing teamwork is Ovretveit's (1997) four-part team analysis framework. Ovretveit proposed that although teams are extremely varied, they can be usefully studied on four dimensions. The four dimensions are:

1   **Level of integration** – Teams can range from loose networks to tight-knit groups where decisions are closely controlled by a collection of professionals.
2   **Team membership** – This dimension is often ignored, but can be very important. Membership of a team of acute care professionals can be quite formal through to very fluid. Membership of a team can also be at different levels, for example full or associate. This may present some difficult decisions, as in, who has full voting rights in decision making, or which types of profession are admitted to the team.
3   **Team process, client pathways and decision making** – This dimension refers to how a service user progresses through a team. It is also about the stages a service user encounters in their 'journey' through the services offered by a team and the decisions that might be made at each of the stages. Ovretveit (1997) describes various types of team: for example, the most common type is the 'parallel pathway team'. This kind of team consists of a separate pathway for each profession. Team meetings are simply opportunities for referral to different professionals.
4   **Team management** – How members of different professions are managed has a profound impact on their effectiveness in working together. Many professionals are managed by members of their own profession up to a certain level, after which they experience general management.

Ovretveit (1997) suggested there are two main challenges when constructing a multi-professional team. One is to create a management system that enables practitioners to have enough freedom in their practice to work most effectively. The second is working out who should be responsible for the overall smooth running of the team as a whole.

Guided Study 5.2

Apply Ovretveit's model of teams to your own experience of an effective or poor team.
Ask yourself about the:

1   **Level of integration**: was your team tightly knit, or a very loose association?
2   **Team membership**: could anyone make a contribution to the team?
3   **Team process**: were there complex arrangements for taking a service user through the process and making decisions about their care?
4   **Management**: was this fair and inclusive?

You could have included:

A range of experiences of teams from your practice, for instance, workplaces we have all known where people hardly talk to each other outside their small groups, and perhaps then only to spread nasty rumours. Other places we may have worked in are very different, being open, friendly environments, where the good feeling extends to people socialising with each other outside work.

(Continued)

(Continued)

Factors such as not allowing health practitioners enough time or space to get to know each other a bit, to start caring for their colleagues as individuals.

Too little or too much change

Rigid, routine-driven, institutional care settings only value obedience; they tend to discourage collaborative team working. In contrast, health care teams can be severely disrupted by constant change, as carefully negotiated plans have to be continually revised.

Factors preventing teamwork in the acute sector

McCallin (2001) reviewed multi-professional working literature, paying particular attention to the teamwork element of multi-professional work. Although she found teamwork was generally poorly defined, and research evidence relatively scarce, McCallin drew several major conclusions. First, teamwork is not in itself the complete answer to providing good quality services. Second, the medical profession dominates multi-professional working in acute health care settings, often to the detriment of collaborative working, though this may be changing. A third conclusion was that conflict between professionals has an enormous negative effect on multi-professional work. On a more positive note, the fourth conclusion from McCallin's review was strong evidence that flexibility in role and good communication were the primary features of effective multi-professional teamwork.

Prejudice

To truly understand multi-professional working, we need to be aware of the positive and negative dimensions of people working together. Professional groupings are like any other collections of people and are prone to the same failings. McCallin's work indicated that discord among professionals greatly reduces the likelihood of effective multi-professional working. A common source of discord arises from different groups of professionals having prejudiced views of each other. Social psychology makes us aware that when groups form, prejudice can follow. Prejudice is an attitude towards an individual or individuals who belong to a group, which is usually negative. Being prejudiced often means disliking a person just because they belong to a particular group, having nothing to do with the real characteristics of the person (Baron and Byrne, 2004). In the everyday world these principles apply to differences such as ethnicity, gender and sexual orientation. In the world of acute health care it could mean, for example, nurses distrusting members of the social work team based on a stereotype, despite the individual social workers being helpful colleagues.

Research has shown that prejudice has several unfortunate attributes, which potentially make it even more harmful to multi-professional working. One of these attributes is that any information relating to an existing prejudice tends to be given more attention. This means that once a prejudice has developed, it can be sustained by paying more attention to it. In addition to this attribute, information that is consistent with the prejudice is more likely to be remembered (Baron and Byrne, 2004). So, for instance, if the members of one profession have a prejudice that another profession is rigid and inflexible, not only will they pay more attention to their responses, but they will be much more likely to remember the times when they were rigid and unbending. Social psychologists have also found that prejudice can be 'implicit', in other words we are often not aware of quite strong biases in our attitudes (Baron and Byrne, 2004). Being unaware of prejudice towards other professionals could clearly make working collaboratively much more difficult.

Social psychologists have proposed a variety of explanations to account for the causes of prejudice, and the main theories tell us a lot about why health professionals in acute care sometimes find it difficult to work together effectively. One of the foremost theories of the causation of prejudice is 'direct intergroup conflict', which suggests that prejudice arises out of competition for scarce, or limited, resources (Baron and Byrne, 2004). All health care services have limits on their funds, and professional groups are in competition with each other to acquire as big a share of the budget, and status, as possible. Another influential theory to explain how prejudice is caused is 'social categorisation'. This approach proposes that we categorise ourselves into groups that are either 'us' or 'them', also known as ingroups and outgroups. We attribute good qualities to the members of our ingroup, the group we belong to, on the basis of their long term, dependable good natures. If members of an outgroup exhibit good qualities, it is temporary, not based on anything substantial (Baron and Byrne, 2004). As you will see later, this idea of belonging to a profession or discipline, and being loyal, is an important factor in multi-professional working in acute care.

The importance of how people behave when placed in different groups, and how prejudice can result, is reflected in research on multi-professional working in acute care. Coombs and Ersser (2004) studied how clinical decisions were made in a UK intensive care setting, discovering two main themes in their findings. The first theme concerned the value given to different types of knowledge by the main professional groups – in this case, doctors and nurses. The medical staff tended to give greatest value to biomedical measures, relegating nurses' concerns with such things as mouth care, skin care and wound care to second best. Intimate knowledge of individual patients and their families was also seen as the nurses' domain, to be drawn on by doctors when necessary. The second theme in Coombs and Ersser's study was the importance of the roles taken by doctors and nurses in clinical decisions, with medical professionals taking the lead. Despite the inconsistencies and limitations of the medical approach to intensive care, the nursing role was simply to comment on the major decisions already made by doctors. These findings suggest an element of the social categorisation approach to prejudice was operating in this situation. The medical ingroup stuck rigidly to biomedical knowledge, only reluctantly using knowledge from the nursing outgroup.

A similar pattern was found by Manias and Street (2001) in a study of critical care ward rounds in Australia. In the ward they studied, rounds had two elements: an initial presentation of patient data in a private discussion room, followed by a lesser element of a bedside discussion. This method was intended to reduce the impact of poor confidentiality and frequent interruptions associated with the traditional full bedside discussion. However, in practice these benefits also led to the almost complete dominance of the ward round by medical professionals. Nurses were 'called in' to the discussion room when their patient was going to be discussed. If the nurse was not immediately available, the discussions largely continued without them and their potential contribution. Contributions made by nurses (as noted in the Coombs and Ersser 2004 findings) were seen as useful, but not as crucial as biomedical measures. The dominance of the medical profession continued in the bedside element.

The practice reported by Manias and Street demonstrates how simple procedures can prevent groups of professionals working together in a collaborative way. The use of a closed room, with doctors controlling entry to the room and the content of the discussions, reinforced historical divisions and hierarchies. The nurses participating in the study made it clear that the ward round method was not deliberately meant to belittle them. However, as you have seen from the findings of social psychology, the forces involved when people are in separate groups are very powerful and not to be underestimated.

Atwal and Caldwell (2006) found similar tensions in their investigation of multi-professional team meetings in three acute care settings: older persons' care, orthopaedics and acute medicine. Nurses from each speciality were interviewed to discover their perceptions of multi-professional working, revealing three barriers that restrained teamwork. The first barrier was the wide variance in what individuals thought multi-professional working meant. This variance included lack of knowledge of the concept itself and scepticism of the value of multi-professional working. A second barrier was the different skills needed to be an effective team member, particularly the confidence required to make a contribution in a multi-professional arena. The third barrier to multi-professional working cited by the nurse respondents was the medical viewpoint dominating interaction in acute care teams. Over-emphasis on the medical contribution was a strong theme in this study, though Atwal and Caldwell (2006) noted that there were distinct differences between the specialities. Acute medical and orthopaedic rounds tended to have little content related to the social history of patients. In contrast to this, multi-professional interactions in elder care actively looked for non-medical social information to inform decisions.

Encouraging multi-professional working in acute care: reduction of prejudice

Atwal and Caldwell's study again found evidence of 'us and them' negative attitudes towards nurses' knowledge. However, the elder care speciality had much less of an 'us and them' approach, showing less prejudice against nursing knowledge. Thus, the finding that not all specialities created divisions demonstrates that ineffective multi-professional working due to intergroup factors is by no means inevitable. Social psychology also researches the conditions for the reduction of prejudice and mistrust between groups. This occurs when groups work cooperatively with each other, learning they are not so bad after all. The simplest method to reduce prejudice and conflict between groups is to increase contact between them, known as the contact hypothesis (Baron and Byrne, 2004). However, contact on its own does not reduce prejudice; it has to occur under certain conditions.

Guided Study 5.3

What factors can help professional groups gain a new respect for each other?

You could have included:

Social psychologists have studied the conditions in which simple contact becomes more positive and reduces bad feeling between groups. A selection is listed below, and may be similar to the ideas you proposed.

- The groups need to be of equal status
- Contact should involve working towards shared goals
- The different groups need to get to know each other as individuals
- There needs to be a culture of group equality surrounding the contact
- People need to think of the other group members they meet as typical of that group.

Therefore, the contact hypothesis provides a model of how health professionals can be encouraged to work together more collaboratively.

No doubt you can easily think of instances in health and social care organisations when groups of people have a lot of contact with each other, but this does not improve relationships between them. Thankfully, though, there are grounds for optimism as professional groups find ways to interact and work successfully together.

A further development of the contact approach in prejudice research is the extended contact hypothesis. Knowing that individuals from your ingroup have successful interactions with members of an outgroup can reduce prejudice (Baron and Byrne, 2004). It has also been found that if two groups come to see themselves as one through some activity that unites them, this reduces mutual prejudice, known as recategorisation (Baron and Byrne, 2004).

Despite the difficulties that are possible in multi-professional relationships, collaborative working in acute health care does frequently occur, demonstrating the prejudice reduction principles just discussed. Studies of multi-professional working in acute care demonstrate that the positive social forces of prejudice reduction can come into play and foster good practice. For example, Scholes and Vaughan (2002) reported on the implementation of new roles in acute care. These new roles were largely those of specialist nurses, carrying out work previously done by junior doctors.

The specialist nurses were initially greeted with suspicion, and sometimes resentment for their 'easy' jobs. This changed over time, as other professionals worked alongside the specialist nurses, growing to respect their expert contribution. Scholes and Vaughan (2002) reported that the initial distrust in many cases changed to positive inclusion into teams, as the new practitioners were used as expert resources. This positive reduction of prejudice was a combination of contact, working towards shared goals, and positive reports of interactions with the specialist nurses.

An example of the kind of specialist practitioner studied by Scholes and Vaughan is the stroke nurse. Burton and Gibbon (2005) studied the benefits to patients of this specialist nurse, who carried out follow-up work with stroke patients and their families, and provided a 'focus for multi-professional working'. Burton and Gibbon's (2005) randomised control trial provided evidence of the benefits to both carers and patients of the specialist stroke nurse.

Guided Study 5.4

Think about a specialist nurse you have come across either through practice placement or giving a presentation in the university. What was their background? What was their expertise and contribution to the multi-professional team?

Need to know more?

Access the following websites to help:

Multiple sclerosis: www.ncchta.org/execsumm/summ517.htm
Rheumatology: www.rheumatoid.org.uk/article.php?article_id=375
Diabetes: www.fend.org/
Cancer: www.macmillan.org.uk
Cardiovascular nursing: www.escardio.org/bodies/councils/CCNAP/

Kvarnström and Cedersund (2006) studied multi-professional health care teams in Sweden. They found that workers all thought of themselves in terms of 'we', which led to successful multi-professional working. There were still difficulties between groups of professionals, but these were lessened because of an open and trusting approach. Kvarnström and Cedersund (2006) also found that this process had to be actively managed, as suggested by Ovretveit (1997), to ensure that the natural divisions between professions did not obliterate collaboration and cooperation. This example shows that prejudice was not allowed to develop in the first place, so workers did not see any important divisions. The frequent use of 'we' to refer to the team was unifying.

Guided Study 5.5

Be honest, there is likely to be some groups of professionals you would rather work with than others! List the groups you prefer and those you least like.

Ask yourself:
What is it about them that influenced your feelings? Social psychology suggests that we like people who are like us. Is this true in your case, or are you responding to a stereotype of particular professional groups? Think back: are there some professionals who you have changed your mind about? What happened to make you change your opinion?

Communication

As noted earlier in this chapter, McCallin's (2001) review of multi-professional working showed that communication (along with flexibility in roles) is very important in fostering good working relations between professional groups. This finding is supported by other sources, along with the converse, that poor communication is a real barrier to worthwhile multi-professional working (Benson and Ducanis, 1995; Birchall, 1997; Burke et al., 2000; Dalley and Sim, 2001). Clearly, communication is vital in all aspects of health care, but has particular features in the context of multi-professional working in acute care settings.

Beringer et al. (2006), in their study of the coordination of children's inpatient services, named communication as the specific factor that contributed most to encourage coordinated working. They also stressed the importance of good quality spoken communication, which allowed for the greater flexibility needed to keep up with constant changes in the children's needs. The disadvantage of this was that staff needed to be in the same place at the same time, and when this was not possible, collaboration was reduced. Atwal and Caldwell's (2006) findings supported this principle, that when particular professional groups were excluded from face-to-face communication, multi-professional working was diminished.

Ensuring the presence and engagement of the whole team in important discussions appears to be vital in ensuring good multi-professional working. Molyneux (2001) studied a successful multi-professional team, working to discharge stroke patients early to benefit from rehabilitation at home. Evidence from this study made it clear that a large part of their success was due to making team meetings a high priority. Attendance by all members and careful consideration of all views were significant features of the quality of collaboration achieved in Molyneux's (2001) study.

It appears that the nature of the communication within multi-professional team discussions is also important, especially given the tendency in acute health care for the medical profession to dominate. Atwal and Caldwell's (2006) participants stressed the need for confidence and assertiveness to prevent their views being ignored. Part of the need for putting views across firmly was to avoid being blamed and humiliated, or as Atwal and Caldwell put it, 'scapegoated'.

The communication within this rather harsh environment contrasts sharply with reports of acute health care teams based on mutual trust and respect. Kvarnström and Cedersund (2006) provide evidence that when a multi-professional team work in an atmosphere of trust, where discussion time is highly valued, there is no need for combative styles of verbal interaction. The outcomes also include direct benefits to service users, as ideas to improve services flow more freely. These findings are supported by other studies. For instance, Scholes and Vaughan (2002) found that effective cross-boundary working was enhanced by team members using personal communication that actively avoided being authoritarian and which encouraged mutual appreciation for other professionals' contributions.

A significant proportion of the findings to do with multi-professional working and communication are concerned with face-to-face verbal interactions. However, some research relates to written information. Molyneux (2001) provides evidence that recording work with service users in central case notes enhances communication between different disciplines. Sloper's (2004) large-scale literature review of multi-professional working supports these findings, promoting the use of shared information, including good IT systems.

Overall, the evidence available makes it clear that discussion between members of different professions involved in an individual's care is vital, and it is especially important for all voices to be heard. It also emerges from the evidence that this sharing of information is even more beneficial to acute care patients when team members have equal status, and trust and respect each other.

Conclusion

In this chapter you have read that the acute care sector has experienced a lot of change in the last few years. A large proportion of this change has challenged traditional professional boundaries, demanding that practitioners cooperate with each other. Our investigation of some examples from acute care practice illustrated this process. Also, examples such as nurse-facilitated discharge and nurse-led VTE services demonstrate how policymakers have often placed nurses in the frontline of multi-professional working.

The evidence explored also makes it clear that teamwork is vital to successful multi-professional working; the membership and structure of teams can be crucial in creating effective acute health care teams. Alongside this, any multi-professional prejudice has to be disarmed to achieve good working relationships. Mutual respect for each profession's contributions and constantly challenging the 'us and them' approach can lead to a reduction in harmful negative attitudes.

However, perhaps the single most important factor in enhancing multi-professional working in acute care is communication. Good quality multi-professional working relies on communication that is open, flexible and includes all views; where all participants have equal status. To combine all these attributes successfully in a multi-professional team presents quite a challenge, but the evidence demonstrates that the effort is ultimately worthwhile: patient care is greatly improved as a result.

PART II

6

Multi-professional Practice and Service Users
Cally Ward

By reading this chapter you will be able to:

- describe the key legislation and policies that are driving change in how professionals work with service users and with each other
- consider the implications of these changes in practice, including partnership working with the people who use services and other professional practitioners
- reflect upon how developments in health and social care policy and practice have the potential to transform radically professional practice in the future.

Introduction

The United Kingdom is currently undergoing a fundamental reform of the whole system of health and social care. This reform will move towards services that are patient and service user led (DOH and British Institute of Human Rights, 2007).

The idea that people who use services should be driving change in public services is at the heart of current public policy. It represents a fundamental shift in the way people who use services are viewed. There has been a shift away from seeing people as passive recipients of services, what has been described as the 'gift model', (Duffy, 2003) to a view of people as citizens who are actively engaged in their own care and support needs, in partnership with those that are paid to support them. (DoH, 2006g). Underlying this is a view that services, and the professionals working within them, will simply get it wrong if they do not involve the people and their families who use these services, at the very heart of the work they do.

This includes the way:

- they work with people on a day-to-day basis
- services monitor and evaluate the quality of what they provide
- that managers strategically plan – and commission – the services of the future.

Nothing about us without us

In 2001, the Government published the White Paper, *Valuing People: A New Strategy for the Learning Disabled for the 21st Century* (DoH, 2001d). This was the first time for 30 years that people with learning disabilities and their families were the focus of public policy in their own right. It represented a milestone in public policy making because it was developed in partnership with people themselves and their families. Valuing People reflected their priorities for change, based on 11 objectives that were set for local services to implement, and were underpinned by a set of four important principles. These principles included acknowledging that people with learning disabilities have the same rights as everyone else and they should be supported to make choices in their lives and be encouraged to be independent and be included in the community. Valuing People made it a mandatory requirement for local authorities to set up multi-agency Partnership Boards to oversee the implementation process, which have to include people with learning disabilities and family carers.

There have been two other significant shifts in health and social care services, which have been explored in detail in Chapters 1 and 3 and are summarised here:

- The first is where care and support is delivered. There has been a move out of institutional settings, like the hospital, into the community and increasingly into people's own homes.
- Second, there has been a shift in the way the role of health and social care is seen. In relation to health, public policy is moving away from a curative concern with 'ill health' to a broader conception of prevention and a focus on health and well-being.

This chapter will discuss the implications of these shifts, both in the way services are organised, funded and commissioned, and the way care and support is delivered. You will also consider the implications these changes have for the way nurses and other human service professionals work with the people they care for and support. You will also reflect on the impact this has on their roles and relationships with other professionals.

Service users and carers – who is it we are we talking about?

Service users

There is no commonly agreed language to describe people who use health and social care services and different organisations use expressions like patients, customers, service users and clients. This lack of agreement is reflected in the way different user groups describe themselves. For the purposes of this chapter we use the term 'people who use services' to cover the range of places that people are supported either in institutional settings or in their own homes.

Carers

The word 'carer' can also cause confusion as it is used in a number of different contexts to mean different groups of people. Most notably we need to differentiate between those people called 'carers' who are paid to offer support, and those people who provide support for other reasons, love, friendship, neighbourliness, a sense of duty or familial obligation and are not paid. These carers are sometimes referred to as 'informal carers' or 'unpaid carers'.

In this chapter, the term family/carer is used to denote the fact that the *majority* of care and support is provided in a family context in people's own homes (although friends and neighbours might also provide care and support and we include them under the heading of family/carer). Many family members find it difficult to relate to the term 'carer' as they see themselves as just 'looking after mum' or in a parenting role, even if these children have reached adulthood (DoH, 2001e; Russell, 2007).

Mutual interdependence

It is also important to recognise that the boundaries between the people who use services and their family/carers are not always clear-cut, especially in an ageing society. There is a growing recognition of the growth of mutual interdependence and care giving and this has important implications for both assessing and delivering support and the way services need to work together (Magrill, 2005).

Partnership with people who uses services and their family/carers: legislative and policy framework

As a student nurse you will be involved in the face-to-face care, treatment or support of your patients, but it is important that you understand the way that legislation and policy impacts on your day-to-day working practices.

The legislative and policy framework is important because it:

* helps shapes the environment where people both deliver and receive services
* shows how people who are in receipt of services and their family carers are perceived by services and treated by the professionals within them

- impacts on the way professional roles and relationships develop in relation to the people they support
- impacts on multi-professional practice as roles and relationships change.

As has been noted, one of the most important policy shifts in recent years has been the emphasis on the involvement of people who use public services in their delivery and design.

The Community Care Act of 1990 was a milestone in that it recognised that you could not just 'fit' people into pre-existing services but you needed to assesses them as individuals and develop tailormade care packages to meet individual needs. At a strategic level the idea of involvement was formalised through the development of Community Care Plans where people who used services and family/carers were seen as key partners in the process (DoH, 1990a).

It is always important to reflect on the purpose of your work, and the organisations you work in, and remind yourself about what it is you are trying to achieve.

> The purpose of service organisations is to meet the needs of customers or service users. Put in its simplest terms, people will get the most from services if those services make sense to them and meet their needs. In order to participate actively, service users need to be engaged in decisions and choices about services and this applies to engagement at every level of the service, whether it relates to an individual drug prescription or setting up a new community resource. (DoH, 2006h: 5)

It is important to distinguish between the different ways people who use services and their families can be involved. All these different ways are important because they influence and interact with one another. For example, what happens at the level of the individual at the point of diagnosis – and particularly treatment – can be affected by decisions made at a local strategic level about financing particular types of treatments. This can be seen in debates about purchasing the drug Herceptin for the treatment of breast cancer and the rationing of the drug Aricept in the treatment of certain dementias.

People who use services are involved at different levels:

At an individual service user or carer level   This is where decisions are made about the services for an individual and their family/carers. The decision making process related to individuals in health and social care is often described as 'assessment and care management' or 'diagnosis and treatment'.

At operational level   This concerns arrangements for service delivery and involvement and could be aimed at helping design a new service, change an existing service or monitor the quality, effectiveness and performance of a service. For example, arrangements to develop a referral system for older people with mental health needs between acute hospital services and the community-based EMI services.

Strategic level   This is the level where decisions are made about the overall objectives and direction of the service development, broad allocations of resources and overarching policy. For example, discussions about the extent to which health and social care services for older people should be jointly managed and have joint budgets. (DoH, 2006i)

Guided Study 6.1

- What happens where you are on placement to involve people in their own care?
- What happens where you are on placement to involve people in evaluating the quality of the service on offer?

Ask some questions in your placement:

- Ask about *how* people are encouraged to work with staff in designing and delivering their support or care plan!
- Ask about *how* the service involves service users and family carers in auditing and evaluating the quality of the service on offer.
- Find out if service users and family carers are involved at senior levels in shaping the *future* development of the services provided.

As well as involving people who use services and their family/carers, there are a number of other key policy themes that have a significant impact on practice, and these themes have been gathering momentum in the last decade. They include:

- The development of person centred practice, where assessment and support is tailored around the need of the individual. You might see this referred to as the 'personalisation' or 'individualisation' of services.
- A shift in *where* care and support are delivered – closer to home.
- The rise of the 'expert patient' and the 'expert carer' – a recognition of the important role that people play in their own care.
- The rise of 'cash for care'. This is where people receive money to purchase their own support rather than being offered or receiving pre-existing services (Glendinning and Kemp, 2006).

In relation to health and social care these key policy themes have been crystallised in the White Paper *Our Health, Our Care, Our Say*, which was published in 2006 after a lengthy public consultation exercise. The emphasis in the White Paper is on empowering people who use health and social services and their family carers to 'make the actions and choices of people who use services the drivers of improvement'.

The White Paper takes a broad view of health and focuses on the idea of delivering a 'health and wellbeing agenda', which aims to achieve the following outcomes for people:

- improved health
- improved quality of life
- an opportunity to make a positive contribution
- an opportunity to exercise choice and control
- freedom from harassment and discrimination
- economic wellbeing
- personal dignity.

In other words, there is an explicit recognition of the role that social and lifestyle factors play in mental and physical health; for example, the impact of poverty, poor housing, or not having a job. These outcomes can clearly only be achieved by effective partnership working between a range of agencies, not just health or social care.

The White Paper makes the following recommendations to help achieve these outcomes:

- resources need to be targeted towards prevention of ill health and social exclusion not just in acute hospital settings
- that people with long-term health conditions need to be supported to manage their own health, with a significant investment in the Expert Patient programme
- there needs to be 'A new deal for Carers' – including developing more emergency breaks, an information line and an Expert Carer Programme and an updating of the 1999 National Carers' Strategy
- more people need to have access to individual budgets and Direct Payments, so they can purchase their own care and support, in the way that best suits them
- more healthcare needs to be delivered outside of hospital
- people should have more choice about where they receive their treatment
- all this can only be achieved through better partnership working across not only health and social care but also housing and other key agencies with these arrangements being formalised through Local Area Agreements. (DoH, 2006b)

The drive to modernise services

Before you leave this section, it is important to consider why these policy changes have come about. These are some factors for you to consider.

Demographic pressure – can services meet the rise in demand?   People are living longer and this demographic pressure has raised serious concerns about the expanding demand for services and the financial pressures on them. These are very real factors and the need to develop support services in this context remains a major political challenge in the future.

However, there are other factors involved in the drive to reform services.

People fighting for their rights – changing expectations   People who use services and their families have a long history of fighting for their right to a get the services that they need. As Colin Goble explains in Chapter 4, people with physical disabilities led the campaign for direct payments. They demanded more choice and control over their support. They wanted to be able to hire their own support workers and plan their own support (Morris, 2006).

This is an example of a policy developing because the people who used services said what they needed and lobbied for it. Although there have been teething problems implementing the policy, and take up has been slow in some areas, direct payments have made a real difference to people's lives (DoH, 2007b; CSCI, 2006).

Family/Carers and their supporters have also successfully lobbied for recognition and support. Over recent years, there have been three laws that have been particularly important to carers:

- 1995 Carers (Recognition of Services) Act
- 2000 Carers and Disabled Children Act
- 2004 Carers (Equal Opportunities) Act.

Because of these three Acts, social services departments must inform carers of their rights. Carers can have an assessment of their own needs and local authorities have been given the powers to provide services to them following a carer's assessment. The assessment must take into account whether the carer works, or would like to return to work, or take up training as well having a break. Social services can enlist the help of housing, health and education to support carer's needs. Family carers can also receive direct payments for support to help them in their caring role.

Commitment to reduce inequalities and anti-discriminatory practice The commitment to reduce inequality and combat discrimination in the last decade is reflected in policy and legislative change (Russell, 2007). It has been driven by recognition that certain groups of people do not enjoy the same life chances as others. Health and social care services do not serve everyone well, as a recent inquiry into the health of people with learning disabilities showed (Disability Rights Commission: Equal Treatment Investigation, 2006). Finding ways of developing services that meet the needs of everyone is now a major priority. Publicly funded organisations have a disability equality duty to ensure that the services they provide can meet the needs of a diverse society. Public authorities also have responsibilities under The Human Rights Act and the Department of Health has published a guide to help health services meet their obligations under the Act (DoH and BIHR, 2007).

Guided Study 6.2

All these things shape the environment you work in and impact on the way you deliver services to the public. What does it mean in your nursing practice?

Think of an example from a recent experience.

Policy into practice

Policy intentions are one thing, making them happen is another. In this section you will look at some of the ways services have changed as result of the changes outlined above and consider the implications of these changes for your practice.

As a health or social professional, you are more like to be delivering care and support in different settings.

Institutional to community and home based care   All the priority community care groups have seen a shift from institutional to community based care since the 1990s, with much greater emphasis on supporting people to live independently in their own homes. This has been accompanied by a greater recognition of the role of family/carers in providing care. There has been an emphasis in acute health services of minimising the length of time people stay in hospital. There has also been the development of the 'intermediate' care for older people to bridge the gap between hospital and home (DoH, 2001c). For more information see Rick Fisher's chapter(3) on primary care.

Assessing people's needs in different ways   In community-based services, the emphasis is on individually based needs assessment. Attempts have been made to simplify assessments into a common, multi-professional assessment framework, and there is within that an emphasis to include self-assessment as much as possible. People are being supported to do this and material has been produced to help carers to prepare to get the best from their carers assessment (Russell, 2007).

Working in partnership with other professionals and their organisations Requirements for better partnership working across health and social services have led to developments in the way professionals are both trained and work together. This has led to the development of some joint professional training courses, the creation of new posts in the health service, new ways of working and the bringing together of professionals and people and their families who use services in shared training initiatives.

Working to involve people who use services and their family carers in their health and social care   Involvement is taking place in different ways. The involvement of people who use services in the assessment of their own needs is now an established part of good practice. The development of Expert Patient programmes (DoH, 2006f) across the country is helping more people to manage successfully their long-term condition, for example, diabetes, and end-stage renal failure. Investment in public health information campaigns like the Obesity programme also plays an important role in trying to prevent long-term health problems (NICE, 2006).

At an operational level, services now find ways of ensuring that the people who use their services are involved in evaluating it, either through questionnaires or through quality audits. There is also evidence that people who use services and their family/carers are more involved in the strategic planning of services (CSCI, 2006).

Working with people who have more choice and control over their care and support   There are a growing number of people who are benefitting from direct payments. The money for people's support needs is paid over to them and they have greater choice and control over *who* supports them and *how* they are supported. The person with support needs becomes the employer. Their supporters are known as Personal Assistants (PAs). Recent developments like the In Control project and the Individual Budget programme take this idea of self directed support a step further by combining a number of different funding streams – not just the care element – to make a reality of the wider health and wellbeing agenda (DoH, 2007c; SCIE, 2007).

Policy into practice – two examples from practice

You are going to consider the implications of the changing policy context for two different groups and look at the implications for professional practice.

Box 6.1 Increasing Choice and Control – Peter's Story

Peter is a 35-year-old man with learning disabilities living at home in Newport with his elderly parents, both of whom are in their late 70s. For many years, Peter and his family have not had any help from services. Peter and his parents did not like what was on offer! But as his parents have got older and developed some health problems of their own it became more and more difficult for Peter to get out and about and for both him and his parents to have a break from one another.

Peter was getting depressed and was having some health problems so his GP referred him to the local multi-disciplinary Learning Disability Team, which included nurses, social workers and other professionals. The community nurse provided him with a health action plan which helped sort out his health issues. The social worker listened to what Peter said he wanted to do in his life and spoke to his parents too, and helped Peter to develop his own Person Centred Plan.

It was agreed that the best way for Peter to get to do the things he wanted to do was to have Direct Payments and employ some local people that he knew to be his Personal Assistants. Peter was able to get out of the house and do the things he liked to do. His parents had some time off caring for him and they were able to enjoy some of the things they liked to do. The Carers Assessment also helped them get some practical help in their own right so they could spend more quality time with Peter when he was at home, instead of worrying about big jobs like gardening. The Community Team also put Peter and his parents in touch with a project, which was helping older family carers plan for the future. Part of Peter's Person Centred Plan was to think about where he might live when his mum and dad died or were too ill to care for him any longer. Peter decided he wanted to stay in the family house and the family were supported in making legal arrangements to do this.

Everyone felt much happier about what was happening in their lives. Peter felt he had a more exciting life and his parents were enjoying having a little more time for themselves. They all felt more reassured about the future as there was a clear plan in place.

Guided Study 6.3

What do you think Peter's story can tell us about some of the important changes in practice and the implications for professionally trained practitioners?

You could have included:

Think about the role of the nurse: are they providing hands-on care or is their role more facilitative? Are they helping Peter and his parents navigate some of the local systems and putting them in touch with organisations that might help, like the Planning for the Future project?

If the role is no longer providing hands-on care, what skills and personal attributes are needed to help people to take more control and have greater choice in their life in the community?

What sort of skills do you think you would need to work effectively in partnership with people who need to use services and their family carers?

What sort of skills do you think you would need to work effectively in a team where there was a mixed group of professional practitioners?

Changes in practice – implications for nurses

Let us turn our attention to another group of people who use services and their families and consider how policy changes are impacting on them. A group of children with complex health care needs have emerged as a result of medical advances (Kirk, and Glendinning, 2004). Government policy to promote home rather than hospital based care has resulted in intensive and specialist nursing care. This is now being carried out in the home by the parents (and sometimes by older children themselves). 'Technology dependent' is the term used to describe children 'who need both a medical device to compensate for the loss of a vital body function and substantial and ongoing nursing care to avert death or further disability' (Wagner et al., 1988: 390) This could include some of the following medical interventions:

- Tracheotomy
- Oxygen therapy
- Mechanical ventilation
- Intravenous drugs
- Parental nutrition
- Peritoneal dialysis
- Gastrostomy.

Developing services to support caring for technology-dependent children at home is not just about transferring medical machinery from the hospital to the home, but it also entails a shift in responsibilities. There is a clear expectation that parents will take on the clinical procedures that have been traditionally done by qualified staff. To do this they will need a lot of information, training and support. It also has important implications for relationships; between children and parents; between parents and staff; and between different groups of professionals (Kirk et al., 2005).

Guided Study 6.4

- What do some of these changes mean in terms of the nurse's role?
- What do some of these changes mean in terms of the skills needed for professional practice?
- What do some of these changes mean for partnership working?

What it means to work in partnership with these children and their families

Working in people's homes requires tact, sensitivity and the demonstration of respect. A home is not a workplace and you need to have the ability to imagine what it might be like if people were marching into your home on a daily basis. How tiring to be 'on show' all the time and feeling that you need to offer to make people cups of tea. This potentially is particularly stressful if you are having agency staff arrive that you do not know very well.

The need to clarify roles and responsibilities

It is important to be clear about your role in supporting or delivering care. It is vital that all the professionals involved have communicated and negotiated their role vis-à-vis one another and the family. Families told researchers that not being clear about the roles of professionals was one of the things they found difficult, and how much they would have valued having roles clarified from the start. This was particularly important when no key worker or coordinator is identified (Kirk et al., 2005).

Educative role: sharing skills and knowledge   When family/carers take on clinical procedures, professionals have an important teaching role. This requires you to be an excellent communicator and be able to support learning and assess the development of technical competence to maintain health and safety and minimise risk. It also means that services need to provide accessible information to support learning.

Sharing caring: the implications of the different knowledge bases underpinning caring for partnership working   Families providing this type of care to their child have to be as technically competent *to care for* their child as professionals are but they also *care about* their son and daughter in a qualitatively different way to practitioners.

This is especially true where there is little continuity in the staff that come into the home. The care that families provide is individualised to their child's needs.

Research indicates that families can be critical of staff for not delivering individualised care based on their child's needs. This is explained by the fact that while family/carers have been trained by professionals and developed technological competence, underpinned by a scientific evidence base, in addition, they also have the experiential knowledge of their child. They are able to respond flexibly to the individual fluctuations of the child's health while the practitioner coming in will not have this knowledge (Kirk et al., 2005)

This can lead to disagreements about the best way to deliver care with both sides making judgements about the others' competence and the child's wellbeing. The potential for conflict between families is perhaps one of the unintended consequences of developing the expert patient and carer programmes.

Acknowledging the emotional impact of caring in a family context It is important for you to acknowledge the emotional impact of caring for those parents who are asked to undertake invasive procedures on their own child: 'The thing I find hard to cope with is that it is my son … and it's seeing him in distress that tears you apart inside' (Kirk et al., 2005: 456). Families need support to deal with a range of potential emotions that come with the responsibility they take on in the care of their child. This includes the fear of hurting their child and the fear of managing risk, and even potential death.

Connecting families to resources and support in the community Families supporting a child with complex needs can feel very isolated (Carlin, 2005). As part of the support you offer the family it will be important to advise them of any support groups they might be able to attend. It will also be important to make sure the parents have a Carers Assessment, which will be their way to access short-term breaks from caring and other support they need. Where there are siblings in the family it would be helpful to tell them about any support groups for young carers that are available in the area so they have some respite from the 'hospital at home'.

All these issues are relevant for your day-to-day practice and are transferable to any other group of people who are being supported to manage long term conditions in their own home.

Moving services forward

It is clear that the future direction of travel for health and social care policy is towards a greater commitment to involve people who use services and their families on a number of different levels. This is reflected in an emphasis on 'individualisation' or 'personalisation' of services and the extension of 'cash for care' schemes like direct payments and the emergence of self-directed support. It is also reflected in the shift in the relationships between 'professionals as expert' to the 'expert by experience'. There is, however, evidence that there is still a long way to go in implementing some of the policy recommendations.

- In a recent choice and equity survey of Primary Care Trusts by the King's Fund, 58 per cent said they had not conducted any assessment to identify who might need support in making health care choices. Two-thirds had not commissioned any new services to support choice (Thorlby and Turner, 2007).
- There is evidence that while people who use services are often consulted about changes, they are often brought in when plans for future developments have already been drawn up. To be effective, and be involved in shaping the agenda they need to be involved fully from the beginning of the process (CSCI, 2006).
- There is concern that people from black and minority ethnic communities are not participating in these processes (SCIE, 2006).
- A recent survey of family/carers of people with mental health needs by the charity Rethink concluded that 'carers were ignored and unsupported' – over half having no regular contact with the staff supporting their family member (Rethink, 2007).
- People benefiting from direct payments have grown in the last five years but the numbers remain small in relation to the majority of people using services. They are currently being developed in social care not health care.
- While there is clear evidence that self-directed support results in positive changes for people and their family the numbers so far also remain small. (DoH, 2007c).
- There is also some evidence that certain groups are less keen to engage with more user driven approaches like direct payments (DoH, 2007c).
- At a local level current financial constraints are putting local partnership arrangements to the test.

Nonetheless, there is a clear commitment to partnership working and a legislative duty to do so. Therefore, the need to address some of these issues does not detract from the fact that the health and social care sector is changing, albeit at a slower pace than policy makers would like.

All these developments will – and are – impacting directly on the roles, functions and responsibility of professionals in some of the ways already discussed.

In terms of your professional practice in the future it is clear that you are likely to be working in a range of different environments, including in the third sector in community settings and people's own homes. Your primary partnership relationship will be with the people you support and their family/carers empowering them to have more choice and control in their lives as they manage their support needs. This focus will also influence the way you liaise with and work with other professionals involved in providing support to people.

Guided Study 6.5

What will this mean for your professional role in the future? What skills and knowledge will you need to work effectively with people who use services and their families in a person centred way?

(Continued)

(Continued)

You could have included:

- A focus on the *capacities* of the people you support and not on their *deficits* as you support them to take more control in planning their support
- You will need to *empower* people through building effective relationships and sharing your knowledge and skills with them
- If you are involved in delivering hands-on care you will do this in a way that is respectful, ensures personal dignity is maintained and is tailored to individual requirements
- You will need to help people to develop specific skills to maintain and sustain their quality of life supporting the development of the expert patient or carer
- In relation to assessment, there is likely to be more emphasis on advocacy and brokerage and less on professional discretion at the point of assessment as you support people and encourage people to self assess
- You will need to work with people and provide them with the tools to *plan their support* in ways that maximise their control and choices
- To do this you will need to help people navigate the systems around them and link them to brokers who can help them *think and plan creatively* about the support they need.

In order to achieve this different type of activity and partnership working, you will need all of the multi-professional knowledge presented in this book – and more – which you will need to learn in practice with feedback from service users and their carers.

Conclusion

In this chapter you have read that, on an individual level, it is clear that the involvement of the person in their own care does have implications for the way you work in practice. What is interesting is that both people who use services and the practitioners that work with them often have a sense of shared frustration when operational and strategic issues act as barriers in developing a truly person centred and flexible support service (Kirk and Glendenning, 2004).

Involvement of people who use services and their families to influence operational and strategic change is less well developed and is the challenge of the future if services are going to be truly personalised. The Department of Health has undertaken a review of public and patient involvement in local services with the view to strengthening arrangements for a louder voice in health and social care (DoH, 2006g). The key points from this are the creation of local involvement networks (LINKs), and a simplifying and strengthening of the duties on health care organisations to involve and consult (DoH, 2006h).

A second element is to look at the way that services are commissioned and to strengthen the involvement of people who use service in this process. The publication in March 2007 of the *Commissioning Framework for Health and Wellbeing* sought to shift the focus of commissioning away from providing services to a focus on improving outcomes. (DoH, 2007d). Emerging research suggests that providing individual budgets to service users, such as people with chronic conditions, can achieve excellent health care outcomes without an increase in costs. (DoH, 2006g).

Although the exact nature of future service provision is not clear, what is clear is that the context of your professional and multi-professional practice will involve working in partnership with the people you support and their families to help them get the support that they need to achieve their health and wellbeing.

7

Nursing and Multi-professional Practice in Mental Health Services
Steve Tee

By reading this chapter you should be able to:

- **identify the key policy, legal and professional framework for multi-professional work in mental health services**
- **describe the key competencies required for multi-professional practice in mental health services**
- **have an understanding and awareness of key skills required to support positive multi-professional work in mental health services**
- **reflect on your own skills for practice and identify where they need further development.**

Introduction

Modern mental health services in the United Kingdom are typically characterised by several agencies working collaboratively to meet the needs of an increasingly complex and diverse population. Mental health nursing is currently the largest professional group working in a range of mental health settings and is considered 'the cornerstone profession' (Jones, 2006: 20). The key feature of a 'cornerstone' is one on which everything else depends. In other words, while the mental health nurse may not always be the lead clinician or agency, they often bind and coordinate activity and generally set the tone for multi-professional practice. Without this cornerstone there will at best be a lack of integration and at worst ineffectual inter-agency and multi-professional practice, leading to potentially dire consequences for the service user.

Over the last two decades there has been a succession of reports into mental health care, often commissioned when things have gone wrong, which cite a lack of multi-professional collaboration as being a significant reason for the breakdown in care. The most well known and, some consider, most significant event in the history of modern mental health care was the killing of Jonathon Zito in 1992 by Chistopher Clunis (Ritchie, 1994). Many others have followed, including in 1996 the death of William Crompton (Crompton, 2007) and in 2004 that of Denis Finnegan (NHS London, 2006). More recently, the National Confidential Inquiry Report (Appleby, 2006) into 'Avoidable Deaths' suggests there have been 400 homicides in the previous eight years by people in contact with mental health services. There is clearly a need for mental health nurses to develop competence in this important area of practice and with this in mind the agency, Skills for Health (2007), has identified a key competence as being able to 'enable workers and agencies to work collaboratively'. In their summary of what this means, which has been mapped against the Knowledge and Skills Framework (DoH, 2004a), Skills for Health state that:

> The workforce competence to work effectively within multi-disciplinary and multi-agency teams is an important dimension in providing effective mental health services. This workforce competence applies to practitioners who have special responsibility within their work role for facilitating collaborative working between workers and agencies ... It is also relevant to those who undertake such a role within agencies through working across a number of practitioner groups. (MH_79, NHS KSFG72)

This chapter seeks to enable the reader, through a process of action and reflection, to examine the skills and knowledge required for multi-professional practice. It begins by exploring the current policy, legal and professional framework for multi-professional work and consequently identifies the relevant competencies demanded of contemporary multi-professional practice. It goes on to discuss key skills using a number of activities to promote deep reflection and develop the readers' insight into their practice.

The context of multi-professional practice

The context of multi-professional practice in mental health is influenced by policy, statutory, and professional drivers which shape the clinical world for the practising mental health care nurse. Awareness of each of these is essential to understand the parameters in which safe and effective multi-professional practice can occur, which in turn seeks to provide the maximum benefit for the service user. To begin the process readers are encouraged to undertake Guided Study 7. 1.

Guided Study 7.1

Reflect on a recent experience in practice of a mental health service user attending a mental health service and record your answers to the following questions:

(Continued)

(Continued)

- Where was the service user receiving care and support?
- What professionals or other carers were involved in providing care or treatment?
- For which agencies did they work?
- Who was leading the care and support?
- What agency was funding the care and support?
- What was the nurse's role?

This exercise will have focused your attention onto the local context in which mental health care is provided. The local context has been arrived at through a national policy agenda, commencing in 1999, which sought to establish national standards in mental health care, of which a key element is multi-professional practice.

The National Service Framework for Mental Health (NSF)

The National Service Framework for Mental Health (DoH, 1999a) has been an important milestone in the modernisation of mental health services in that it established a long-term strategy for the standards and provision of contemporary mental health services. An External Reference Group was established to develop ten guiding values and principles to shape future decisions on service delivery written from the perspective of people experiencing mental health problems.

Box 7.1 NSF Guiding Values

- Involve service users and their carers in planning and delivery of care
- Deliver high quality treatment and care which is known to be effective and acceptable
- Be well suited to those who use them and non-discriminatory
- Be accessible so that help can be obtained when and where it is needed
- Promote their safety and that of their carers, staff and the wider public
- Offer choices which promote independence
- Be well coordinated between all staff and agencies
- Deliver continuity of care for as long as it is needed
- Empower and support their staff
- Be properly accountable to the public, service users and carers
- Reduce suicides.

No single agency can achieve these standards alone and implicit within the principles is the need for professionals providing care to work together and ensure a well coordinated and accountable service. Following the publication of the NSF, the Government issued a series of Policy Implementation Guides (PIGs), which supported the delivery of mental health policy locally. The first overarching guide was published in 2001 (DoH, 2001b), followed by specific guidance relevant to the clinical specialties listed in Box 7.2.

Box 7.2　Policy Implementation Guides (PIGs)

- Adult Acute (DoH, 2002f)
- Community Mental Health Teams (DoH, 2002g)
- Dual Diagnosis (DoH, 2002h)
- National minimum standards for general adult services in Psychiatric Intensive Care Units (PICU) and Low Secure Environments (DoH, 2002i)
- Support, Time and Recovery (STR) workers (DoH, 2003b)
- Community Development Workers (DoH, 2004e)
- Learning and development toolkit for the whole of the mental health workforce across both health and social care (DoH, 2007g).

Copies of the PIGs can be found at: www.dh.gov.uk/en/Policyandguidance/Healthand socialcaretopics/Mentalhealth/DH_4031694

In order to deliver such radical change the emphasis has been on local health and social care communities working together to plan for implementation of the new models of service delivery. Coordination is the watchword with recognition that such a comprehensive programme of change cannot be achieved by a single agency or a single profession working alone. It is acknowledged that a defining characteristic of an effective mental health service is the involvement of a range of disciplines planning the care of a single individual which should include:

- suitable accommodation
- adequate income
- meaningful occupation
- family support
- competent diagnosis, treatment and care.

This reforming agenda also emphasised the need for services to communicate across functional and geographical boundaries to ensure criteria, referral systems and protocols were both coordinated and complementary. This change emphasised a whole systems approach, with Local Implementation Teams (LITs), first established in 1999, working to implement the NSF in their area (DoH, 2001a). LITs are seen as inclusive bodies with representation from health and social care, statutory and voluntary sectors, professionals, service users and carers. LITs were required to take a root and branch look at systems to support new service patterns. A key requirement has been to ensure the availability of sufficient staff with the right competencies, who reflect the diversity of the local community and who can work in a multi-professional context. Important outcomes of this work have seen the development of new and innovative community services including:

- assertive outreach
- crisis resolution
- early intervention teams.

The policy drivers have had far-reaching effects on the shape of mental health services, although some continue to argue that the drive for reform must continue, particularly in the area of the legal framework in which treatment and after-care is provided which, it is suggested, has not kept pace with service reform.

The legal context of multi-professional practice

This section does not seek to provide a complete account of UK mental health law but focuses on elements particularly pertinent to multi-professional practice. In England and Wales, the Mental Health Act 1983 is the most significant, but increasingly outdated, piece of mental health legislation that makes provision for the compulsory detention and treatment in hospital of those with mental disorder. The Act also focuses on after-care and makes it clear that the central purpose of all treatment and care is to equip people to cope with life outside hospital and function successfully without danger to themselves or others. It is further suggested that the planning of multi-professional after-care should begin on admission to hospital. In many ways this emphasis exposed an issue for service providers in that mental health legislation has not kept pace with evidence based practice and service reform. To address this, the current UK Government has introduced a new Mental Health Bill (DoHk, 2006).

Mental Health Bill

The Mental Health Bill (DoH, 2006k), and consequent Mental Health Act (2007), has important implications for multi-professional practice, in that it seeks to ensure that people with serious mental disorders can be required, where necessary, to receive the treatment they need to protect them and others from harm. It is suggested that this will be achieved through amending the 1983 Act to simplify and modernise the definition of mental disorder and the criteria for detention and to introduce supervised community treatment. It is anticipated that the new Bill will bring mental health legislation into line with modern service provision by allowing a broader range of professionals to carry out functions, currently within the 1983 Act, and by enabling people to be treated in the community where appropriate. The Bill also aims to strengthen patient safeguards and tackle human rights incompatibilities. While some of these reforms are considered controversial and remain subject to considerable debate among professional bodies and mental health lobbying groups, it is likely that the Bill will further shape the mental health nurse's role. In parallel with these legal reforms, the nurse's role, and that of other disciplines, has also been shaped by the evolution of a framework for the delivery of community care known as the Care Programme Approach.

The Care Programme Approach (CPA)

The Care Programme Approach (Department of Health 1990b, NHS Executive and Social Services Inspectorate, 1999) (see Box 7.3) was introduced in 1990 and revised in 1999, to acknowledge the reality that most mental health care was provided in the community. The CPA is the framework for good practice in the delivery of mental health services and was a response to concerns that community care, for both formal and informal patients, was poorly organised with a lack of clear accountability and responsibility. A recent report on the CPA, undertaken by the Sainsbury Centre for Mental Health (2005), stresses the need for staff from all disciplines and agencies to work together to ensure continuity of care between hospital and community settings. The CPA provides a framework to ensure community services are coordinated and work well together and requires professionals from the health authority, local authority and other agencies to arrange care. There are currently two sub-domains to the CPA, namely standard and enhanced.

Box 7.3   Care Programme Approach

- Systematic arrangements for assessing people's health and social care needs
- The formulation of a care plan which addresses those needs
- The appointment of a key worker to keep in close touch with the patient and monitor care
- Regular review and, where necessary, agreed changes to the care plan.

Standard and enhanced CPA

The difference between the standard and enhanced domain relate to the level of involvement and support the service user will need and whether there is any element of risk to themselves or others. While it can be seen from the criteria for the domains (see Box 7.4) that multi-professional practice is intrinsic within both, it is a more significant aspect of enhanced CPA, which places greater demands on those with responsibility for coordinating care.

Box 7.4   Criteria for the Levels of CPA

Standard CPA

- Require the support or intervention of one agency or discipline
- Require low key support from more than one agency or discipline
- Be more able to self-manage their mental health
- Have an informal support network
- Pose little danger to themselves and/or others
- Be more likely to maintain contact with services.

Enhanced CPA

- Multiple care needs, including housing, employment etc, requiring interagency coordination
- Willing to cooperate with one profession or agency, but have multiple care needs
- May be in contact with a number of agencies (including the Criminal Justice System)
- Likely to require more frequent and intensive interventions
- More likely to have mental health problems co-existing with other problems such as substance misuse
- More likely to be at risk of harming themselves and/or others
- More likely to disengage with services.

Care coordinator

The decision as to who should take on the care coordination role is an important one and should be determined by local protocol, taking account of professional issues, the views of the service user and local agreements. In reality the role is normally undertaken by one professional, usually a nurse or occupational therapist, but sometimes a social worker, psychiatrist or psychologist. The care coordinator will remain in regular contact with both the patient and their carer(s) and will arrange a regular review of the care plan to both ensure care is being delivered and to negotiate changes. It is the care coordinator's responsibility to send a copy of the written care plan to all professionals involved, including the individual's GP.

The written care plan should address an individual's social, medical and nursing needs. Care-planning meetings commonly take place before the patient is discharged from hospital and will involve the patient and, with agreement, their family or other carer. The agreed care plan is then shared with the professionals involved on a need to know basis. The CPA process and the coordinating role are important responsibilities for mental health service providers and are enshrined in section 117 of the Mental Health Act 1983. This requires health and social services authorities, in collaboration with the independent sector, to provide after-care for certain categories of detained patients. It is further stated that after-care of detained patients should be included in the Care Programme Approach and that before the decision is taken to discharge or grant leave to a patient, the responsible medical officer, in collaboration with the other professionals should assess the patient's needs and ensure the care plan fully addresses them. A helpful guide detailing the role of the care coordinator can be found at: www.dh.gov.uk/en/Publicationsandstatistics/Publications/PublicationsPolicyAndGuidance/DH_4009221

The nurse's role

It is clear that mental health nurses have a key role in the planning and coordination of a person's after-care, a significant element of which is to ensure that the right people are present at the planning meetings. Section 27.8 of the Code of Practice provides a useful checklist (See Box 7.5), although many providers have developed their own checklists to reflect new service structures and agencies involved.

Box 7.5   Code of Practice: Section 27.8

- The patient, if he or she wishes and/or a nominated representative
- A nurse involved in caring for the patient in hospital
- A social worker/care manager specialising in mental health work – the GP and primary care team
- A community psychiatric/mental health nurse
- A representative of relevant voluntary organisations
- In the case of a restricted patient, the probation service
- Subject to the patient's consent, any informal carer who will be involved in looking after him or her outside hospital
- Subject to the patient's consent, his or her nearest relative
- A representative of housing authorities, if accommodation is an issue.

It is evident that the responsibility for planning and coordinating care places significant demands on the practising mental health nurse. These demands – set alongside the legislative changes reported above and the modernisation of mental health services – suggested it was timely to undertake a root and branch review of the mental health nurse's role.

The Chief Nursing Officer's review of mental health nursing (Department of Health, 2006) – 'From Values to Action'

Within the CNO review it was acknowledged that the majority of mental health nurses work as part of a multi-professional team. It emphasised that this was a time of great change in mental health for professional roles and relationships between the various professions, which demanded considerable skills in advanced communication and coordination, as well as understanding and respecting others' perspectives. It was also made clear that in order to adhere to their code of conduct, mental health nurses may at times have to assertively put forward their views regarding the best interests of service users, even if this challenges the views of others within the multi-professional team. The review adds that this requires strong leadership to promote effective and confident nursing practice within the multi-professional setting.

What are the key competencies for working multi-professionally?

What emerges from the CNO review and the policy, legal and professional parameters previously outlined, is the need to identify and develop a range of skills and competencies which support multi-professional practice. In the field of mental health, to a great extent this has been the focus of the Sainsbury Centre for Mental Health (2001), who developed the Capable Practitioner Framework. According to the Sainsbury Centre (2001), capability includes a performance component which identifies the 'what', an ethical component which integrates awareness of culture and values, and a reflective component concerned with learning in and from practice. It is further suggested that this should all be underpinned by evidence-based interventions and a commitment to lifelong learning. As a consequence of this work the Sainsbury Centre Joint Workforce Support Unit and the National Institute for Mental Health in England (Hope, 2004) developed the ten essential shared capabilities, which are a framework for the whole workforce.

The ten essential shared capabilities for mental health practice (Hope, 2004)

It is stressed that the ten essential capabilities (see Box 7.6) do not replace but complement other competence frameworks by providing the mental health specific context and achievements for education and training at pre-registration stage.

Box 7.6   The Ten Essential Shared Capabilities for Mental Health Practice

Working in partnership   Developing and maintaining constructive working relationships with service users, carers, families, colleagues, lay people and wider community networks. Working positively with any tensions created by conflicts of interest or aspiration that may arise between the partners in care.

Respecting diversity   Working in partnership with service users, carers, families and colleagues to provide care and interventions that not only make a positive difference but also do so in ways that respect and value diversity including age, race, culture, disability, gender, spirituality and sexuality.

Practising ethically   Recognising the rights and aspirations of service users and their families, acknowledging power differentials and minimising them whenever possible. Providing treatment and care that is accountable to service users and carers within the boundaries prescribed by national (professional), legal and local codes of ethical practice.

Challenging inequality   Addressing the causes and consequences of stigma, discrimination, social inequality and exclusion on service users, carers and mental health services. Creating, developing or maintaining valued social roles for people in the communities they come from.

Promoting recovery   Working in partnership to provide care and treatment that enables service users and carers to tackle mental health problems with hope and optimism and to work towards a valued lifestyle within and beyond the limits of any mental health problem.

Identifying people's needs and strengths   Working in partnership to gather information to agree health and social care needs in the context of the preferred lifestyle and aspirations of service users, their families, carers and friends.

Providing service user centred care   Negotiating achievable and meaningful goals; primarily from the perspective of service users and their families. Influencing and seeking the means to achieve these goals and clarifying the responsibilities of the people who will provide any help that is needed, including systematically evaluating outcomes and achievements.

Making a difference   Facilitating access to and delivering the best quality, evidence-based, values-based health and social care interventions to meet the needs and aspirations of service users and their families and carers.

Promoting safety and positive risk taking   Empowering the person to decide the level of risk they are prepared to take with their health and safety. This includes working with the tension between promoting safety and positive risk taking, including assessing and dealing with possible risks for service users, carers, family members and the wider public.

Personal development and learning   Keeping up-to-date with changes in practice and participating in life-long learning, personal and professional development for one's self and colleagues through supervision, appraisal and reflective practice.

Source: Hope, R. (2004) *The Ten Essential Shared Capabilities – A Framework for the Whole of the Mental Health Workforce.* Department of Health, NIMHE, SCMH Joint Workforce Support Unit.

The ten essential shared capabilities clearly emphasise the need for effective multi-professional practice through its emphasis on partnership working, challenging inequity and ethical practice. For instance it would be difficult to respect an individual's diverse background without being mindful of the need to work closely with other community agencies and professionals. Equally, the promotion of recovery demands multi-professional interventions which achieve a valued lifestyle for the individual. No one professional group will have a monopoly on all the answers.

Achieving capability towards multi-professional practice

This next section will draw on elements of the ten essential shared capabilities (Hope, 2004) and identify key skills required for effective practice. It is, however, not practical to learn all that is required from a book. Learning will be enhanced through immersion in multi-professional teamwork followed by reflection on experiences gained in practice, such as the following activity.

Guided Study 7.2

Reflect on a recent experience of communication within a multi-professional mental health team.

Identify aspects of your experience you enjoyed. What made it enjoyable?
Identify aspects of the experience in which you felt less comfortable. What made you feel uncomfortable?
Describe the characteristics of the communication patterns between the different professionals involved.
In what ways do you think communication between the professionals could be improved?

Communication in multi-professional practice

In completing this exercise you may have found yourself reflecting on an excellent experience of multi-professional working in which there were high levels of dialogue between professionals, mutual respect and harmonious relationships.

More commonly, you may have had a mixed experience in which there were examples of effective communication but also situations where communication was lacking and perhaps where you felt uncomfortable due to the way some professionals regard each other. This was an issue encountered by a student, which was reported in a study into teamwork:

... well I had this pep talk from Bob (manager) and nothing matches what was said ... staff are really despondent, the consultant is an arrogant s***, and some staff hate each other's guts ... thank God all teams aren't like this or I'd jack it tomorrow. (Stark et al., 2002: 411)

Typically, multi-professional teams only function effectively when participants within the team are prepared to invest the time and energy to make them work. Communication is essentially an interaction between people. While there are many other texts written on the subject of communication, in the context of multi-professional practice it can achieve a number of functions. These may include obtaining or conveying information, expressing one's own needs or those of a client, developing an understanding of each other's roles or acting assertively where there is a need to take control of a situation. It is also the tool used to develop trust in our relationships with other people. Arguably, effective multi-professional practice will only occur in an environment where there is clear, open and transparent communication between individuals and organisations.

Communicating within a multi-professional environment requires similar skills to those adopted when working with clients; for instance, the ability to establish empathy and to develop rapport. The nurse needs to behave assertively and with confidence and to be able to convey a professional and proactive approach. On occasions the nurse may need to be persistent to ensure their voice – and more importantly that of the client – is heard.

Challenging self-limiting beliefs: understanding our values attitudes and beliefs

Understanding your values, attitudes and beliefs is important, as they affect the way you behave and the decisions you make. The personal and professional attitudes and values you hold can both enhance and hinder effective multi-professional working. An attitude is simply a feeling or opinion about something or someone, whilevalues tend to be more deeply held convictions which influence our behaviour. Awareness of both is important for working together and agreeing priorities and needs.

Mental health nurses need to become aware of their attitudes and values about other professionals so that they do not negatively influence decisions. Some examples of the attitudes suggesting openness toward multi-professional practice in mental health are identified below:

Box 7.7   Attitudes

- Respect for other professionals and their beliefs
- Desire to see professionals working together in a positive way with service users' needs and preferences being at the centre of service delivery
- Valuing of diversity and of different perspectives
- Upholding the right of all professional groups to contribute to the planning of care
- Adopting a proactive approach to multi-professional practice
- Ensuring the safety, health and well-being of professional colleagues
- Treating people with respect and dignity and where necessary observing their right to privacy and confidentiality.

This list is not intended to be exhaustive and you might want to add your own examples. However, the important point is that awareness of your attitudes, values and beliefs can be developed by first reflecting on your practice with other professionals and then checking out the evidence for our beliefs. Sometimes people hold stereotypical views of other professionals which turn out to be wrong. Stereotypical views can cause us to behave in prejudicial ways and may inhibit working relationships. For instance, if you have had a bad experience communicating with a social worker you may go on to carry the belief that 'all social workers are the same'. This may lead you to avoid sharing important information and putting others at risk. It is therefore necessary to identify your beliefs about others so that you can overcome potential sources of prejudice and avoid negative consequences. Consider the following activity.

Guided Study 7.3

Liam is a service user living in Belfast. Liam has a diagnosis of schizophrenia and receives visits from a community mental health nurse. Liam also has regular contact with a social worker, psychiatrist, occupational therapist and support time and recovery worker.

1 List on paper what you believe to be the core activities and responsibilities of the professionals identified in the scenario.
2 Ask professional colleagues undertaking similar roles what they see as their core activities and responsibilities and also record these on paper.
3 Compare your lists and highlight differences.
4 Identify any areas of overlap.
5 Were there any surprises arising from this exercise?
6 What are the implications of the areas of overlap and how can these be managed?

Working collaboratively and in partnership

In order to develop harmonious working relationships it is helpful to consider the notion of partnership. Partnerships include relationships where individuals or groups work in mutual cooperation and responsibility. In the mental health practice setting, partnerships will be established within the context of social, political, cultural, legal and familial issues affecting the service user. For example, where an individual requires a package of care provided by a number of agencies from health, social care and the independent sector, these will need to be clearly identified in the form of a written care plan, with the operationalisation of the agreed package founded on the principles of partnership.

Some have made the distinction between multi-disciplinary or multi-professional care and inter-disciplinary care (Berger, 2006), suggesting that the prefix 'inter' implies synthesis of practice with mutual collaboration and agreement of outcomes. However, in reality, working practice is dependent less on terminology and more on professionals' attitudes toward partnership working, and in this book writers have stressed the use of the term multi-professional as fundamental in partnership working. To appreciate the implications of partnerships for practice it is worth noting Towle and Godolphin's (1999) partnership principles, which imply:

- mutual responsibility where all involved make a contribution
- debate and agreement about the relationship between those involved
- an organic process which can adapt to changes in circumstances
- a relationship which can begin at anytime and which needs time to develop.

These considerations are important as they emphasise that multi-professional practice requires commitment of time and resources and provide a potential diagnosis when multi-professional practice appears to be going wrong.

While the ideal conditions for partnership working are mutual respect and shared decision-making, unfortunately such processes also provide opportunities for some professionals to dominate proceedings. This is a real and important issue as, if not acknowledged, it can impact on the mental health care received by the service user, as well as the morale of the team. Handy (1990) highlights how in professional relationships a power imbalance can arise as a consequence of a person's position in society:

> ... systematic distortions by dominant power holders whose structural position in society gives them an enhanced ability to make their own sectional interests appear to others as a universal one. (1990: 359)

While the 'systemic distortions' referred to here can arise from many sources and need to be tackled, it is probably unrealistic to expect that, in future, multi-professional mental health practice will take place within an egalitarian environment where everyone is acknowledged as equal and all contributions are considered with equanimity. However, sadly, too often the use and misuse of power can be observed in the dynamics of professional teams and needs to be challenged, to enable authentic communication to flourish. While such behaviour may simply arise from beliefs that different professionals hold about what other professionals do, which Nolan (1993) argues will influence how practitioners work together, such behaviour is less likely to occur where there is a high level of trust, empathy and genuineness occurring across disciplines. To be effective the mental health nurse needs to be alert to and appreciate power differentials so that they can identify them, work with them and where necessary challenge them. Such action will help to avoid disempowerment of both the nurse as a professional, with an important contribution to make and, more importantly, the person receiving the service.

Building trust in multi-professional practice

Overcoming power differentials and building authentic working relationships requires trust. Building trust is a multi-faceted process whereby participants can either enhance or erode trust through action or omission. Awareness of our beliefs about multi-professional practice helps us avoid premature judgements and behaviour which may impede the development of an effective trusting partnership. Trust, between professionals, takes time to build and is too easily broken through insensitive communication. The skills used in building relationships with clients, such as active listening, empathy and promoting meaningful dialogue, will serve the nurse well. Such skills help to facilitate communication and develop insight and understanding into each other's perspectives, thus building respect.

Where professionals can achieve mutual respect and dialogue there is a much greater likelihood of a successful outcome for the service user. However, as in any relationship, where an individual believes they are being ignored, misunderstood or manipulated this will damage trust and could have consequences for the care being provided. Avoiding such an outcome requires sensitivity to the way others work. Rogers (1970) identified three core conditions which he suggested were necessary for relationships to be productive:

1   Empathy: Being able to view the world from the perspective of another person and to reflect it back so that the other person can hear it. Achieving empathy within multi-professional practice does not mean that you necessarily have to agree with their view, but it does require the skills of attentive listening and expressing appreciation of the others position in order that one can negotiate common ground.
2   Acceptance: Trust requires acceptance so that people can explore their differences. Also known as unconditional positive regard, acceptance acknowledges people's value irrespective of their view of behaviour. However, importantly this does not mean approval or admiration of another's position but is an important mindset in which everyone is regarded as equal.
3   Genuineness: Genuineness requires honesty and integrity. It means behaving without façade and avoiding adopting an 'expert' role.

Learning from each other through active dialogue

Providing the core conditions outlined by Rogers (1970) are present then it is more likely that sensitive and productive dialogue can occur. According to Isaacs (1999), dialogue is a conversation which does not take sides and which avoids vested interests. Thus it is through active dialogue between professionals and agencies that networking and learning happens. Senge (2006) adds that dialogue enables groups to explore multiple perspectives, while suspending preconceived notions.

Through such dialogue a process of co-created and shared meaning occurs and by drawing on the contributions of many disciplines and professionals, support for a particular endeavour will develop. The mental health nurse plays a crucial role in contributing their knowledge of the bio-psycho-social aspects of mental health and of local services, but also through listening to others and responding sensitively. An example of this may be discussion around the care of someone with a dual diagnosis and the need for mental health and learning disability services to work in partnership in order to meet a client's diverse needs. However, as Onyett points out, partnership will amount to nothing if it does not achieve strengthened collaboration requiring:

inter-agency care planning and assessment where providers meet to assist service users … there needs to be inter-agency ownership of decisions to commit resources to meet the wide range of needs of individual users and their carers. (2003: 70)

Planning care together

Planning care together requires considerable skills of facilitation towards action oriented solutions. Many care planning initiatives fail because there is a lack of clarity about the goals to be achieved, the timescales to be observed and the person(s) responsible for taking the actions. An important consideration when planning care is who should be involved. Multi-agency approaches to care planning require engagement of those agencies who will participate in an individual's care. However, large meetings with many professionals may be daunting for service users and so consideration needs to be given to the potential impact on service users and how this can be effectively managed while maintaining their involvement in the process. An important consideration is to ensure that care is focused on the needs of the user rather than the needs of the professional. Considerable strides are being made in many services in the use of wellness recovery action planning (WRAP), which adopts a client led approach to care planning (Copeland, 1997).

Whatever the approach taken, it is important not to underestimate the importance of this process for multi-professional, multi-agency and client engagement, which will ultimately determine the success or otherwise of the package. The mere process of promoting active dialogue between professionals can be an important leveller, bringing professionals into closer contact with alternative perspectives and, importantly for the mental health nurse, interventions being set in the context of the expressed needs of an individual and/or their family.

Guided Study 7.4

Planning Care Together

You have been asked to coordinate a multi-professional ward round and clinical review. What practical arrangements would you make to ensure that the service user and family members were able to contribute?

The team assembles and includes, a consultant psychiatrist, SHO, two ward based nurses, a social worker, two community mental health nurses, a psychologist, an occupational therapist and two community support workers.

How would you ensure that all group members were able to contribute to the discussion?

After an initial presentation and discussion the team deliberates over the care plan.

How would you ensure actions are captured and recorded?

How would you end the group discussion?

Managing conflict in multi-professional mental health care

Of course, any group of people working together raises the potential for conflict. Achieving a position where priorities are agreed may not be a straightforward journey. Those leading participatory approaches will benefit from an understanding of Tuckman's (1965) framework for determining the progress of team development. Tuckman suggests that teams will work through stages that he called forming, storming, norming and performing. Being aware of these stages will help the nurse to expect and respond appropriately to behaviours at different stages of the group's development.

Facilitating a multi-professional group meeting

Where a group of professionals come together for the first time, according to Tuckman (1965), there will be a tendency to be overly polite, often with superficial interactions and an impersonal atmosphere, which may lead to some inhibited behaviour. The skills required will be those that help the group feel comfortable with each other and may include some initial introductory exercises, sharing expectations and agreeing group rules. During this stage the facilitator will get a sense of the commitment to the group and sense any potential areas of dissent.

As group members familiarise themselves with each other, 'storming' behaviour may arise during which participants will challenge each other and perhaps even want to withdraw. This is perhaps the most important stage of the group as skilled facilitation can either support or inhibit effective collaborative working. Facilitation skills will be those that encourage dialogue and openness and ensure equal contributions from all participants. The skills of summarising, reflecting and paraphrasing will be key as they will help to ensure that points of view are acknowledged and respected.

Once the storming stage has been successfully navigated, positive group norms will emerge which enable open and transparent dialogue, allowing conflict to be managed productively. The facilitator's role is directed at building and promoting the positive norms and facilitating toward potential solutions. A key outcome is to be able to facilitate the decision-making process toward consensus rather than domination by one particular group, individual or special interest.

The final stage of performing is where participants collaborate effectively within an atmosphere of authentic participation. At this stage the facilitator's role becomes easier but no less crucial in maintaining the group dynamic towards action oriented solutions with agreed responsibilities, timescales and dates.

The above model can apply to groups which run over several meetings or for a one-off meeting, but of course the timescale for negotiating through the different stages will be different. Whatever the size or duration of the group meeting the key skill is that of sensitivity to the evolving atmosphere of the group and contributing to an atmosphere of trust, hope, safety, appreciation and respect.

As previously indicated, multi-professional working needs to put the service user at the heart of its decision-making as it has the potential to become subverted into a professionally oriented decision-making process rather than user oriented process. Large multi-professional groups, while essential for collaboration and shared agreement – and essential for effective mental health care – may not be the most user-friendly approach to decision making. One way of enhancing a user focused approach is to involve an advocate who can participate on behalf of an individual or group.

Advocacy in multi-professional mental health care

The process of advocacy involves:

> Either an individual or group with disabilities or their representative, pressing their case with influential others, about situations which either affect them directly or, and more usually, trying to prevent proposed changes which will leave them worse off. (Brandon et al., 1995: 1)

Mental health nursing practice should ideally seek to promote autonomy and self management through recognition of the individual's strengths and capability. However, it is sometimes necessary to advocate on behalf of individuals or groups, particularly those considered vulnerable, to ensure their rights and interests are safeguarded. Advocacy may be necessary in care planning situations where a person cannot express their own needs or are intimidated by large groups of professionals.

Guided Study 7.5

What advocacy agencies are available in your area?
How are service users informed of available advocacy services?
What are the arrangements for involving advocacy services in planning care?
What considerations should be made when involving advocacy services in the care planning process?

There are likely to be many instances where individual service users are experiencing severe mental health symptoms, such as cognitive impairment, which affects their ability to take an active role in treatment and care decisions. In such cases ready access to an advocate may enable them to participate and ensure their voice is heard. Therefore effective multi-professional practice is that which facilitates free and open access to advocacy agencies and promotes their involvement in the care planning process.

Record keeping for multi-professional practice in mental health

There has been an understandable preoccupation with the quality of record keeping in nursing for professional and legal reasons (Caldwell et al., 2000; Nursing and Midwifery Council, 2006). While the principles of good record keeping are common to all fields of nursing, the Nursing and Midwifery Council (2006: 1) make the point that it is a professional practice tool to support the care process and as such is: 'not an optional extra to be fitted in if circumstances allow'.

They go on to suggest that effective record keeping provides for improved communication and dissemination of data and information between professionals and, as such, it is key to multi-professional working. In mental health it is increasingly common to have a single patient record, with integrated systems between health and social care providers, thus aiding communication across organisational boundaries. It is the nurse's responsibility to support this system by ensuring accurate factual records, which includes a record of any advice given by other professional colleagues.

Leadership in multi-professional mental health practice

An important element of multi-professional practice in mental health is the need for skills in leadership in terms of setting direction and having a clear purpose. Such qualities are consistent with those of a transformational style of leadership (Dawes and Handscomb, 2005). Despite policy and legislative expectations nurses may encounter variable commitment to multi-professional working among different agencies. As coordinator of care the nurse will need to encourage and motivate. This might mean appealing to higher ideals and moral values and being able to articulate a clear vision of what the multi-professional involvement is aiming to achieve (Mullins, 2007). The effective leader will also recognise the interpersonal impact of making change and will seek to provide individualised support to professional colleagues.

Conclusion

This chapter has shown that multi-professional practice in mental health requires an investment of time and the commitment to make it work, as well as the skills to facilitate effective collaboration. Collaboration also needs to be driven by a determination to ensure the values of service user-oriented decision-making are central to any multi-professional process. Developing an appreciation of effective practice cannot be achieved at a distance. It requires nurses to immerse themselves within the day-to-day practices of multi-professional teams in order to develop insights into professional roles, key networks and potential resources. It is the nurse who leads and understands organisational systems and dynamics that can bring about greater integration between agencies and improve the outcomes for their clients. Perhaps the greatest lesson to be learnt is the realisation that clients' problems are often so complex that no single agency can provide all the answers. Consequently, it is the nurse who can work flexibly and across traditional boundaries who is most likely to realise the outcomes that are valued by the clients they serve. Janet McCray will explore leadership further in the final chapter of this book.

8

Nursing and Multi-professional Practice in Children's services
Sandra Wallis and Janet McCray

By reading this chapter you should be able to:

- consider the key drivers for change in multi-professional working in children's services
- describe the legislation and policy drivers to support these changes
- reflect on the likely impact of this legislation on professional roles and multi-professional practice
- work through case studies which will enable you to develop your understanding of multi-professional knowledge and skills for this challenging area of practice.

Introduction

Nowhere in the delivery of public services has the quality of multi-professional working received more public scrutiny or censure than in services for children. As a result, a number of organisational and professional failings have been highlighted in the numerous public inquiries that have made uncomfortable reading. In children's services a powerful driving force towards collaborative work has been in the field of child protection. Here, more than in any other area, the impetus to do better is enforced through policy documents which are far reaching in terms of strict guidance for professionals working with children.

As a student nurse you may well have observed early in your community experience the level of collaboration and community engagement of health visitors and midwives with other disciplines from a range of services supporting children and families. Some of these relationships are in well-established networks and of long standing. Other relationships and accountabilities are new, and set within a wider agenda in relation to outcomes for children and families. The challenge for all professionals is to make these new links and emerging networks a success, at the heart of which are the quality and extensiveness of the multi-professional relationships in place.

Let's look first at the origins of current changes.

Legislative frameworks

The Welfare State, as it is now known, was first introduced in 1946 after the then Labour government's success in the post-world war two general election.

The government set up Children's Departments alongside the other major changes. The first of these departments were quite small and were relatively un-hierarchical by today's standards. It was recommended that the newly created Children's Officers should be women, because of their 'maternal' knowledge of childcare. With some minor changes this remained the position until the 1960s when major changes to children's services were introduced.

The Seebohm legislation in the late 1960s marked the beginning of a period of unprecedented change in the whole structure of local government in England and Wales. Children's Departments, Mental Health and the Welfare Services provided by local government were subsumed into Social Services Departments. A few months later this was followed by local government boundary changes. These resulted in hitherto Unitary Authorities losing out to enlarged County Councils that led on to the creation of large bureaucratic organisations. Scotland enacted separate legislation by way of the Social Work (Scotland) Act 1968. Part 12A. www.scotland.gov. uk/Topics/Health/care/ Joint Future/Publications/SWS12A/Q/f accessed March 11, 2008.

It was around this time – as huge and costly changes were in train – that the first of the series of 'modern' child abuse scandals occurred when Maria Colwell was killed in Sussex (Colwell Report, 1974). A report of the Tonbridge Wells Study Group (1973) identified key areas of failure across the professions, highlighting inefficient procedures in communication systems, administration, planning liaison and supervision (McCray, 2003: 12). One response to these findings was the issuing of guidance around the coordination of child protection. Further developments occurred with the Court Report (DoH, 1976), which was to establish multi-disciplinary teams and the start of integrated child health services.

There have been numerous enquiries since the death of Maria Colwell in 1973. One of the findings from this inquiry was the lack of communication between the agencies involved with Maria's family. Unfortunately, this lack has been noted repeatedly in many of the reports of inquiries that have followed. Inter-agency changes were recommended as a result and this led to the setting up of Area Review Committees and Child Protection Registers as part of the development towards working more closely together to protect children. Nevertheless, failures in coordination have continued throughout the past three decades and further recommendations followed later inquiries, such as those into the deaths of Jasmine Beckford (Blom-Cooper, 1985) and Tyra Henry (London Borough of Lambeth, 1987).

In 1989, The Children Act was brought into being so as to modernise the whole area of legislation surrounding children in both the public and private sectors. Biggs (1997: 190) notes the Children Act 1989 (DoH, 1989a) and the report *Working Together under the Children Act 1989* (DoH, 1991) clarified the arrangements for multi-professional working across the professions which were to be demonstrable. The most recent and far-reaching inquiry has been that which investigated the circumstances surrounding the death of Victoria Climbié (Laming, 2003). The Government's response to this tragedy was the introduction of the Children Act 2004 and the policy agenda *Every Child Matters*. The White Paper and resulting legislation has had a far reaching impact – not least the break up of Social Services Departments into Adult Services and Children Services. The split has placed Adult Services firmly within the Health arena while those of Children's Services have been placed under the umbrella of the newly designated Department of Children, Schools and Families.

At the heart of all these developments has been the need to address public concern for the protection of children perceived to be at risk.

In health care, a public inquiry into children's heart surgery at the Bristol Royal Infirmary between 1984 and 1995, chaired by Professor Kennedy, had discussed the need for a broadening of professional competence and recommended a number of actions in relation to communication, respect for the perspective of other professionals and a need for more multi-professional education. The subsequent development of the National Service Frameworks for Children, Young People and Maternity Services, starting in 2001, were also as a result of the reforms following the inquiry into the death of Victoria Climbié.

The Change for Children programme incorporated the National Service Frameworks for Children and set out the government's plans for an integrated service for pregnant women from birth through to adulthood with ambitious national standards set. The standards are in three parts: standards 1–5 for all children; standards 6–10 for children with complex needs or circumstances; and standard 11 which refers to maternity services (DoH, 2004f). Nurses, because of the breadth of their professional role, are likely to be working with other professionals to achieve all of the standards relating to their place of work. For example standard 7 refers to children who are in hospital, affecting acute care nurses; while standard 10 is linked to medicines so may involve nurses who are qualified as nurse prescribers in community or primary care settings. This bringing together of agencies who had previously worked separately was formalised in legislation.

The publication of the White Paper *Every Child Matters* in 2004 (DFES, 2004) and the new Children Act (2004) underpin this different perspective on children's needs. Fundamental to the implementation of *Every Child Matters* is inter-agency partnership under the statutory requirements of section 10 of the Children Act, which sets out arrangements for local health care trusts, local authorities and the voluntary and independent sectors to work together in the commissioning, design and delivery of services, for children and young people in children's trusts (DFES, 2005). This Act introduces a requirement to cooperate. Section 10(2) states that:

> The arrangements are to be made with a view to improving the well-being of children in the authority's area so far as relating to:
>
> a) physical and mental health and emotional well-being;
> b) protection from harm and neglect;
> c) education, training and recreation;
> d) the contribution made by them to society; social and economic well-being.

Previously a greater degree of cooperation was encouraged – it is now enshrined in law.

These changes mean radically different ways of multi-professional working for all professionals – from the strategic leader to the practitioner in the frontline. They reflect the government's shift in emphasis in terms of taking action not just to prevent child abuse, but to bring together their key aims around tackling childhood poverty, creating inclusion and integrating their health, education and welfare. It is perhaps here in the provision of children's services that these far reaching policy aims are starting to becoming reality. The next section will look at their intended impact on children and young people.

For all of the agencies involved with children it is *Every Child Matters* (ECM) that is currently setting the agenda. Here, the five 'outcomes' introduced by ECM are:

- Be healthy
- Stay safe
- Enjoy and achieve
- Make a positive contribution
- Achieve economic well-being.

At first reading they may seem to be quite ordinary outcomes, but they do include all aspects of what 'good' parents want for their children. They also, quite cleverly, bring together all of the agencies required for their achievement – Health, Children's Services, Education, Employment and Careers, Police and Leisure.

The Laming Report of 2003 made 108 recommendations – many quite general – but the numerous specific recommendations (numbers 64–90, for example, relate to health services alone) have produced an enormous amount of literature affecting all professional groups. The detailed recommendations to try to improve practice include, at number 72:

> No child about whom there are concerns about deliberate harm should be discharged from hospital back into the community without an identified GP. Responsibility for ensuring this happens rests with the hospital consultant under whose care the child has been admitted. (Para. 9: 105)

The Government's continuing response to the report was *Every Child Matters: Next Steps* (DfES, 2004), which described the new legislation as 'the first step in a long term programme of change'.

We ought to conclude this section with a tacit recognition that the many legislative provisions that successive governments have put forward in response to the numerous public inquiries into child abuse over the years have not thus far led to their elimination. Nor, according to the Laming report (2003), have the agencies involved been able to exhibit the kind of joined-up working that has long been recommended. Indeed, according to this report, many of the practices that would have alerted the agencies involved to the plight of Victoria Climbié were already in place, but were simply not carried out. Hospital staff did not report suspicious injuries; frontline workers failed to make visits and available information was not shared.

One explanation for the problems around multi-professional information sharing is in the differing professional cultures of Health and Children's Services. It has been suggested that patterns of information sharing may be influenced by a number of factors, including not only multi-professional differences in the approach taken to information sharing but also the ways in which the professions interrelate (Richardson and Asthana, 2006).

Impact on service provision

Such a major blueprint for transformation means that children's services should be comprehensively joined up and inclusive. Yet as you have seen, in some areas of provision children and their families have been let down at critical times of transition in their lives. For example there are gaps in services when young adults with a disability or a learning disability move from full-time education, to further education or in children with disability from birth to five years before they start nursery and school. The government report *Aiming High for Disabled Children* (DFES, 2007) sets out where services are failing children and young people and what needs to be done to address these shortfalls. The report notes a lack of coordination across agencies in relation to 'different eligibility criteria; differing referral systems and cultures, and differing and inconsistent data about the disabled children population across agencies' (DFES, 2007: 23).

What happens for children and families is often in response to a crisis rather than planned and integrated service provision. Because health services do not register disabled children at birth, they rely on often inadequate data about how many children with a disability they need to provide services for. Social care agencies assess and collect data on those families and children who are registered, but do not necessarily inform other agencies. From a family perspective this may mean constantly being assessed by different professionals for separate needs, resulting in no overall planning and access to a range of disparate and often uncoordinated services. As a nurse you may be working directly with the family coordinating assessments, but you could also be leading strategic projects to change local provision in the light of poor reviews of your current local provision. Good practice tells us that development of new and user centred services require agencies and organisations to work together at all levels.

The Care Service Improvement Partnership (CSIP) sets out the two crucial factors for more integrated delivery of services. These are good information when planning services and the need for improvements in the way people work together to gather information and interpret it (CSIP, 2007). The CSIP has produced a self-assessment audit tool to support service improvement, based on the National Service Frameworks for children, young people and maternity services standard eight, which is aimed at children and young people with complex health needs. This tool is designed to help local agencies gather information, identifying gaps in service for disabled children and their families, using accurate data. Significantly, the tool can enable better collaborative working as it provides a framework for agencies to use to work together. In order to make this happen the CSIP suggest that commissioners of services should be involved, and that key managers from agencies are identified to lead their part of the service change. This is important, because all too often poor multi-professional practice occurs because those seeking change do not appoint a clear leader with vested authority. In a study by McCray (2003: 119), one nursing participant describes her frustration when working multi-professionally: 'You expect social care agencies to take accountability and be supported by their senior managers when the reality is budgets and numbers.'

Likewise, social workers may be critical of nurses who expect the lead professional role in a team project to stay in social care, even when this is not stipulated in any guidance or legislation.

It is also important to know your local context well. Open systems thinking (Iles and Sutherland, 2001) tells us that change cannot take place if parts of that system are isolated. In reality all systems and the processes within it are interconnected. To create real change all parts of a system should be involved in identifying the change and how to make it happen. Let's look at this in relation to services for disabled children. If you were unaware of other agencies and professionals involved in offering support in an area, you might exclude them from planning strategies to design new services. So it is important to seek the views and networking information of other agencies and professionals, otherwise you would be continuing to contribute towards plans offering services based on poor information, while perpetuating the disjointed and poorly coordinated services you are trying to replace. Equally, you may assume that another agency or professionals are providing input when this is not the case. Consequently, a gap in service could occur and a child may be at risk. So taking into account all aspects of care and its delivery are vital for positive change to happen for families.

Guided Study 8.1

What multi-professional knowledge is required of the nurse who is involved in integrating children's services?
At practice level?
As a project leader?

A good working knowledge of the major requirements of ECM is needed at both levels.

At practice level

- You need to know how and where to contact your local Safeguarding Children Boards – these have been set up as a result of the new legislation (replacing the one time Area Child Protection Committees).
- Prior to any child protection meeting you attend you should ensure that you have:

    1 given yourself sufficient time and opportunity to read up on the details of the case and discuss it with your project leader
    2 tried to update your evidence base in relation to the particular case being dealt with (by consulting your project leader, other colleagues and/or accessing relevant articles in professional journals/books)
    3 worked out the contribution you will be able to make at the upcoming child protection meeting. This could be the considered view of what your particular health expertise can bring to the situation and you should be prepared to defend it.

- In dealing with a particular case you should also be ready to 'think outside of the box' to see whether, for example, there may, in this case, be some organisational structures present that could actually work so as to prevent what seems to be best practice.
- Try to get into the habit of reflecting on the outcomes of your cases to see in what way you may be able to improve on your presentation and advice in any future meetings.

As a project leader

As a project leader you should try to provide the context at practice level which allows your practitioners the opportunity to participate fully in the decision making processes and help equip them with the confidence to assert their professional opinion regarding the cases they deal with.

Need to know more? Chapter 9 of this book exploring multi-professional leadership will help you.

Vulnerable children

As noted earlier, the scope of changes to children's services are far reaching, joining up traditionally segregated services so that vulnerable children do not fall through the net of support available. The government's intention is to identify and respond proactively to the needs of those children and families who may – with additional intervention – avoid family breakdown and potential abuse. Equally, the government is concerned at the inequality of opportunity for all children and particularly for those in care. One example of support for parents and children is the Sure Start programme which aims, as Malin and Morrow (2007: 457) note, to offer 'early and sustained support for children and can help them succeed at school and help reduce crime, unemployment and teenage pregnancy and other social and economic problems'.

At this stage, it seems it is too early to assess the effectiveness of this initiative (Carter et al., 2007a). This kind of preventative role, however, does not just lie with Sure Start, as it now forms part of the brief of all services supporting children.

A number of other initiatives underpin and support this. Notably *Quality Protects* (DFES, 1999) and *Every Child Matters: Change for Children in Social Care* (DFES, 2004). These emphasise the integrated nature of all parts of service delivery from assessment through to the commissioning of services. Key dates were set to achieve Common Assessment Frameworks (CAFs) to prevent children being at risk due to gaps in service. The CAF is to be used by all agencies to integrate the data and avoid repetitive assessments. Funding to provide services is linked to the achievement of specific targets. The CAFs are important because they promote early assessment across different services, with their aim of promoting the sharing of information and using a formal evidence base for identifying vulnerable children. In theory, agencies should no longer work in isolation but share data and information from very early on about children and their situation. This CAF process should identify children who have complex or additional needs and require the support of an additional professional, who will coordinate the input of a range of professionals for children who have multiple needs. Nurses are able to take on this role, which should be determined by the nature of the child's situation. However, if the child is at risk of abuse it is likely that the social worker who will have statutory responsibility will take on any additional lead professional responsibilities.

The social work role in child protection is underwritten by legislation. Section 47 of the Children Act 1989 gives statutory responsibility to Children's Services to investigate children at risk in their area. The lead professional role, while having family-focused advocacy skills at its centre, involves multi-professional practice skills and knowledge.

Guided Study 8.2

What multi-professional skills would a lead professional role require of the nurse?

You could have included:

- Strong communication skills, including diplomacy and sensitivity to the needs of others
- An ability to establish effective and professional relationships with colleagues from different backgrounds

(Continued)

(Continued)

- An ability to convene meetings and discussions with different practitioners
- An ability to translate their own knowledge and understanding into effective practice
- An ability to work in partnership with other practitioners to deliver effective interventions and support for children, young people and families
- An understanding of other key professionals, and how to contact them for consultation or referral
- Knowledge of local and regional services for children and young people, what they offer, and how to contact them.

Source: www.everychildmatters.gov.uk/deliveringservices/leadprofessional/skills knowledge/

A number of other qualities are identified in the *Every Child Matters* guidance (DFES, 2005), including personal characteristics. Jumaa (2005: 162) cites Goleman (1998), who suggests that good leadership requires emotional intelligence, which includes good social skills:

> Handling emotions in relationships well and accurately reading social situations and networks, interacting smoothly using these skills to persuade and lead, negotiate and settle differences for cooperation and team work. (Golemann, cited in Jumma 2005: 318)

In the often stressful and crisis-driven arena of Children's Services this is essential, while a further quality, that of 'acceptance and respect from other practitioners in relation to the role and functions of the lead professional' (DFES, 2007a) is vital. Good multi-professional working is often dependent on the credibility of the professionals involved. Not only does the lead professional require their own skills and knowledge, the DFES notes the need for 'Clear and transparent systems developed and agreed at strategic level, in relation to line management, accountability, professional support, and escalation routes' (DFES, 2005).

From an individual perspective, it is essential when taking on such a role that you are clear about your own management, have set in place your clinical supervision and know how to gain support from above you in the organisation if there are major or urgent crises to resolve.

Putting knowledge into practice

As you can see new forms of service and multi-professional working require new knowledge and skills for all professionals. The following case studies will help you consider what you need to know to be an effective professional in children's services.

Case study A

Guided Study 8.3

Rose Maddox is a 32-year-old pregnant woman who has been known to mental health services for a number of years. Rose has misused drugs since she was 17, and has been homeless and living on the streets in the past. The Probation Service has since found her accommodation. She is five months into her pregnancy and she has been referred to Children's Services by the mental health team for a child protection conference because of concerns about her lifestyle and the possible effect on her unborn child.

Make a list of as many professionals and others as you can think of who might be involved.
How would you work with them?
What would you expect your contribution to be?

Rose (it is essential that the service user's perspective is central in any assessment)
Rose's family
GP and Health Visitor and Midwife
Mental Health
Housing
Probation
Children's Services: (Threshold for entitlement is Section17 of the *Children Act 1989*)

a) Family Support (including Family Centres) and disabled children
b) Looked after children (Section 20 of the *Children Act 1989*)
c) Child protection (Section 47 of the *Children Act 1989*)
d) Adoption and Fostering Services (*Adoption and Children Act 2002*).

With regard to how you would work with them, note that there are likely to be communication issues. There could, for example, be different agendas between Probation, Health and Children's Services – Probation concerned with drug misuse; Nursing professionals with the welfare of both mother and child (midwife, community nurse, health visitor); and the Children's Services professionals in their child protection role may be mainly concerned about the unborn child.

Not all work with children and families may be as crisis-focused as Rose's situation – but it could be equally complex. As you will have seen from reading this book, a number of other cases may also require multi-professional collaboration. Think about a different situation you have been involved in for case study B.

Case study B

As you work through this exercise we hope you have been able to identify when multi-professional practice worked, as well as where it could have been better. If there were issues around accountability or roles a review of Chapter 7 may also help you, while Chapter 6 sets out some of the ways of working that user-led practice requires and will support you to further think through your role in the situation you have explored.

Conclusion

This chapter has shown that even if you have yet to work with children and families, often such work is stressful, potentially involving conflict and almost certainly requiring the application of a number of multi-professional skills, knowledge and values. For most professionals – including nurses – children and family work is practised at a later stage in their qualifying career. However, you could be a student nurse in A&E at an early point in your career and be faced with a potential child at risk scenario, so it is important to be developing the multi-professional knowledge and formal communication strategies introduced here at whatever stage in your career you are at.

This chapter has also offered you some further sources of information for you to take forward into practice. We hope this will enable you to become confident in your skill and knowledge preparation for work in this challenging but important area of multi-professional practice.

9

Nursing, Multi-professional Practice and the Third Sector
Terry Scragg

By reading this chapter you should be able to:

- **define what is meant by the third sector**
- **describe the historical development and current role of the third sector**
- **assess the changes in the role of the third sector and the impact on multi-professional working**
- **reflect on the impact of these changes for the NHS and the new professional and multi-professional partnerships emerging.**

Introduction

The third sector is a significant provider of health services, including acute treatment, residential and nursing care, and palliative care. The sector has become a key partner in the provision of health and social care services under the modernisation agenda of successive Labour governments. This chapter will begin by defining what is meant by the third sector, followed by an explanation of how the sector has evolved from the early charitable provision established prior to the NHS. It will then provide definitions of the terminology used in the third sector, and the development of third sector organisations in health care. You will see how the provision of services is changing as a result of policies that support a growth of health provision provided by third sector organisations. In view of the increasingly important role this sector plays in health care it is critical that you understand the sector, its policy framework and how effective multi-professional working relationships can be forged with organisations working in partnership with the National Health Service (NHS).

Defining the third sector

The term 'third sector' embraces a wide range of organisations, including charities, community and voluntary organisations and other not-for-profit and civic organisations whose primary objectives are social rather than economic. The third sector distinguishes all these organisations from the 'private sector' and the 'public sector'. Furthermore, they share two common characteristics; unlike private sector organisations they do not distribute profits to their owners, and unlike public sector organisations they are not subject to direct political control. They have the independence to determine their own future (Hudson, 2004). Third sector organisations are seen to provide distinct benefits, including closeness to those who use services, strong community links and local accountability, flexibility and freedom from control, innovation and resourcefulness in the use of resources and planning (Bubb, 2003).

The voluntary and community sectors

Within the third sector, voluntary organisations are enormously diverse, ranging from small local community groups providing a service to a specific group of service users through to large national charities that are household names, such as Help the Aged and MENCAP, with structures and processes that mirror large public sector organisations. The main feature of voluntary organisations is that they exist to promote social, environmental or cultural objectives for the benefit of society as a whole or particular groups within it. They are independent of government and public services and are self-governing. They are value-driven and non-profit making, with certain tax advantages, re-investing any surpluses in the development of services, rather than distributing profits to shareholders. They must meet strict conditions about their overall purpose and set up a constitution for purposes of governance. They are funded in a variety of ways, including donations from the public, payment for services (for example on contract from the NHS and local government), government grants, legacies or trading, such as charity shops. In 2006 the sector had an income of £26.3 bn, with 600,000 people employed in the sector, equivalent to 488,000 FTEs (full-time employees), with a growth of 20 per cent in the last ten years. As you have seen, the sector is very diverse with 90 per cent having an annual income of less than £100,000 (NCVO, 2006).

The history of third sector provision

There is a long history of voluntary hospital services in the UK, with many having their roots in the charitable response to poverty and ill health in the Victorian age. Historically, charitable and voluntary hospitals were a key part of health care before the introduction of the NHS, although some of these were selective and dealt mainly with serious illnesses, alongside municipal and private provision. For example, the Royal Free Hospital began as a charity in 1828 to provide free hospital care to those who could not afford health care, whereas St. Bartholomew's and St. Thomas's hospitals have an even longer history dating back to the twefth century. The weakness of this system was that coverage and quality varied from area to area, with access to services dependent on a person's ability to pay or reliant on the charity of doctors who gave their services free to the poorest patients, with significant sections of the population having no access to health care. The introduction of the NHS in 1948 meant services were free at the point of use, with the state becoming the monopolistic provider of health care. This has been changing gradually since the market reforms of the Conservative governments of the 1980s and continues as part of the Labour government's modernisation agenda for the NHS, with the trend of greater involvement of independent sector providers (private and voluntary) in health care provision mirroring wider changes in society. In housing, the vast majority of social housing is now provided by third sector housing associations. Similarly, over 40 per cent of social care services are now provided by the private and voluntary sector. In all areas of social policy third sector organisations are a growing element in the provision of services, moving from the periphery to the mainstream of service delivery.

New alliances and partnerships

With the growth in patient expectations and means of empowering patients, the NHS is increasingly drawing on the third sector. The report *High Quality Care For All* (DoH, 2008b) sets out its vision for more partnerships between the NHS and the third sector, whilst *Putting People First*, a shared vision and commitment to the transformation of adult social care (DoH, 2007h), further affirms the central focus on personalised care and partnerships between the NHS, statutory social care services and the third sector. Many of these developments are in the very early stages as this chapter is being written. Current examples include the 'Expert Patient Programme' (www.expertpatients.co.uk), designed to give people more confidence, skills and knowledge in managing their health condition more effectively in order to improve the quality of their lives, and the Princess Royal Trust for Carers (www.carers.org), which is similarly supporting the development of expert carers. This growing confidence in the third sector is reinforced by a recent statement from the Commission for Social Care Inspection (CSCI) that services run by voluntary organisations significantly out-perform both local authorities and the private sector (CSCI, 2005). Labour governments have seized on these third sector strengths, as witnessed in the establishment in 2006 of an Office of the Third Sector (OTS) with a Minister for the Third Sector, who has stated that 'the third sector has strengths in innovation and engaging with service users which are lessons for the statutory service, and transforming public services through third sector delivery and drawing on third sector skills' (the *Guardian*, 20th September 2006). The Office will also coordinate the work of other government departments, including establishing a Public Service Innovation

Team, whose work will include building an intelligence bank of third sector good practice. The Office has also published a cross-governmental action plan and is committed to the long-term programme of support to the third sector.

Types of organisations in the third sector

There are a range of terms used to describe services provided by not-for-profit organisations delivering health care, either in terms of local community groups or larger charities providing services on contract to local government and the NHS. The third sector increasingly describes a range of organisations which are neither state nor private sector, including small community groups, large established national and international voluntary or charitable organisations.

Voluntary and community sectors

This includes charities registered with the Charity Commission, as well as non-charitable non-profit organisations, associations, self-help groups and community groups. Most involve some aspect of voluntary activity though many are professional organisations with paid staff. Community organisations tend to be focused on particular localities or groups within the community, and many are dependent entirely or almost entirely on voluntary activity. In 2006 there were around 168,600 registered charities, and in additional several hundred thousand small community groups.

Social enterprises

These are businesses with primary social objectives whose surpluses are reinvested for that purpose of the business or community rather than being driven by the need to maximise profit for shareholders and owners. This is a growing area of development in health care as the Labour government see social enterprises as a means of reinvigorating health service delivery, using business models within a not-for-profit value base. In 2005 there were around 55,000 social enterprises.

Cooperatives and mutuals

These cover a wide range of organisations, based on the values of self-help, democracy and equality, which include consumer, worker, agricultural and housing cooperatives. In 2005 there were over 8,000 registered societies. An additional group of organisations that are part of the cooperative and mutual movement are the 567 credit unions, which are financial services societies with half a million members.

> ### Guided Study 9.1
>
> You should now have an understanding of the main features of third sector organisations, and may even have direct experience either in a personal capacity or through your professional studies. From what you have learnt so far try to answer the following question.
>
> **What do you see as the main features of third sector organisations?**
>
> You will have found that third sector organisations are value-driven, commonly share social, environmental or cultural objectives, and that they are independent from government and reinvest their financial surpluses for those same objectives.

How third sector organisations work

Legislative framework

Voluntary organisations are registered and regulated by the Charity Commission, which is a non-governmental department, answerable to Parliament. There are separate arrangements in Scotland and Northern Ireland. The Commission offers support and guidance to the sector, including training and information on the governance of voluntary organisations. Currently the sector is controlled by the Charities Act 1993, but this has recently been replaced by the Charities Act 2006, which was implemented gradually over the last two years. This new Act is intended to simplify the administration of charities and reduce the regulatory burden, particularly on smaller charities, including the exemption from registration for some very small charities. Other provisions include making it easier to merge charities and to simplify the auditing regime for charitable companies. It also provides a clearer definition of a charity with emphasis on its public benefit role. The Act will also modernise the Charity Commission's functions and powers as a regulator of the sector, and preserve its independence from government.

Scotland   Scotland also has a new piece of legislation in the Charities and Trustee Investment (Scotland) Act 2005. This set outs a comprehensive regulatory framework for third sector organisations in Scotland. Scotland also established under the Act the Office of Scottish Charity Regulator (known as OSCR, www. oscr.org.uk), which acts as the statutory regulator for the sector. Scotland has an active charity sector of approximately 18,000 organisations.

Northern Ireland   A new charity law, The Charities (Northern Ireland) Order 2007 is expected to take effect in late 2008 (www.opsi.gov.uk accessed March 11, 2008). It will establish a Charity Commission for Northern Ireland and create a new register of charities. The new act will introduce for the first time a statutory definition of a 'charity' and a list of charitable purposes similar to that found in the English legislation.

Strengths of the third sector

Why is the government so keen to encourage the third sector to provide health services? The basis for change is the view that the traditional public sector is too centralised, top-down, unresponsive and inefficient. Although the critique of state provision began with the Conservative governments of the 1980s – with the introduction of markets for health care as a means of challenging state provision – since 1997 the Labour government has continued to emphasise the importance of 'what matters is what works, not the delivery mechanism'. This is the view that a plurality of providers, including the third sector, is thought to drive up standards and increase choice, which is encouraged by government. The specific advantages of the third sector are five fold:

- The sector is seen to deliver services that are closer to service users, including engaging service users in the design and delivery of services that demonstrates a local accountability that is more responsive and bespoke delivery.
- Many organisations have strong community links and local accountability, particularly the potential to articulate the voice of citizens and service users who find that state services are inappropriate or inaccessible.
- They provide the potential for entrepreneurship, including fundraising, networking and finding innovative solutions to intractable problems, which is increasingly demonstrated in the social enterprises that are now growing rapidly.
- Third sector organisations are generally seen as less bureaucratic than public sector organisations, and therefore avoid some of the barriers to change and slow response to new demands found in public sector organisations, and by the very nature of their funding need to be resourceful in the deployment of staff and other resources. This demands more flexibility in roles and relationships than found in traditional public sector organisations and enables the third sector to respond quickly to new demands and requirements.
- Third sector organisations are credited with the ability to innovate, with many of the issues now addressed by government departments and the statutory sector shaped by the actions of third sector organisations who turned tolerated conditions into problems and claims for action. It is this potential for action that makes third sector organisations attractive to politicians seeking solutions to social problems (ACEVO, 2004).

Concerns about third sector development

In spite of a wide range of statements about the third sector's ability to provide services that are more responsive, innovative and flexible, there has been little detailed research on the performance of the sector, with a lack of robust data to support the statements made by third sector leaders. In one of the few studies of third sector delivery of public services, focusing on user experience, the National Consumer Council (Hopkins, 2007) researched three services (employment services, domiciliary care for older people and social housing). The findings of this research suggested that it was not possible to generalise about public services delivered by third sector organisations due to the distinctiveness of the services and the different delivery models employed. The research did find that the third sector was distinctive in delivering employment services, whereas there was less distinctiveness in its delivery of domiciliary care and social housing services. In domiciliary care services the private sector was found to be significantly more responsive to service users and in housing services there was little to choose between local authority managed housing and housing associations. Commenting on this research Benjamin (2007: 2) states that the 'NCC report punctures some of the unhelpful hype around third sector capabilities, but also highlights the paucity of evidence on which the government's love-in with the voluntary sector is based.'

A further area of concern is the increasing polarisation of the third sector between large national organisations operating as government contractors, and smaller organisations engaged in a struggle for shrinking amounts of funding according to the Public Administration Select Committee (PASC) which launched an inquiry into 'the growing trend towards government buying and commissioning services from the third sector' (Public Administration Select Committee, 2007a). Issues of concern to the committee included the risk that the sector's independence is becoming compromised by its contractual relationship with government and questions about how 'contracted out' providers of public services can be held accountable. The Select Committee developed a series of questions that probed the costs and benefits of the government's policy on the third sector. Question included, whether the third sector is able to provide better public services that the state or private sector; the impact of commissioning on the third sector and the financial implications of providing services through the third sector compared with state provision. The response of the review (Public Administration Select Committee, 2008) showed that there was no evidence that the third sector delivers distinctive services, such as specialist knowledge or expertise than other sectors, with much of the evidence hypothetical or anecdotal. Nor did the evidence suggest that the sector is more innovative, or that the third sector had higher or lower standards. Although this was partly down to the difficulties of assessing performance levels in public services. This view is important when value for money is a key factor in commissioning services, and was seen as critical to effective third sector organisations. The committee used the term 'intelligent commissioning' with scope to involve the third sector more, fostering an understanding of the sector's strength among commissioners in the NHS and social care who are central to determining the shape of public services.

A third area of concern, and one which the third sectors leaders have identified (Bubb, 2007: 17), is the risk of 'incorporation', where larger organisations take on the bureaucratic forms of public sector organisations and 'become less interested in innovation and less able to respond flexibly to new challenges or unmet need'. These concerns are mirrored by the Charity Commission's concerns that charities delivering public services are more likely to be affected by 'mission drift' or pressure from funders and less likely to involve trustees in decisions about what activities they will undertake (Charity Commission, 2007). In the drive to secure contracts and expand the range of services provided by third sector organisations there are risks that organisations will be so transformed by their new role that they in turn are seen as bureaucratic and unresponsive and come to resemble the statutory services they have been encouraged to replace. The growth of voluntary and community services, contractual relationship with the state risks undermining the level of trust between organisations and the public, with a tension between 'doing good' in the ethical sense and 'doing well' in the organisational sense. If trust is eroded this may undermine individual's willingness to participate in voluntary and community services (Tonkiss et al., 1999).

Third sector policy developments

Current policy developments originated under Conservative governments of the 1980s with changes in public services intended to reduce the role of the state and encourage the development of service delivery by non-governmental organisations, including the private and voluntary sectors. Many of the current changes have their origin in the reforms of the period 1987–1990, when the Conservative government introduced its White Paper *Working for Patients* (DoH, 1989b), later enacted as the NHS and Community Care Act 1990. These reforms created the internal market, separating the funding of services from their provision, challenging the power of hospitals and giving GPs the power to purchase services. The reforms created the 'mixed economy of care', consisting of state, private and voluntary sector provision of health and social care services. Although these market based changes were subsequently reformed by the Labour government with the introduction of the 'Third Way', the main thrust of reforms have continued with a series of policy initiatives that have led to a growth in third sector and private provision of health services.

In 1998 the government (Home Office, 1998) published its Compact (www.policy hub.org.uk) on relations between government and the voluntary sector, which acknowledged that the government and the sector had distinct – but complementary – roles and highlighted the value of working in partnership towards common aims and objectives. In 2004 the government introduced the Strategy Agreement between the DoH, NHS and voluntary and community sector, to give the voluntary sector a more central role in supporting and providing NHS services (DoH, 2004g). This is intended to increase capacity and widen patient choice. The intention is that this strategy will promote and support joint working at local level through innovative partnerships. More recently, the government produced a guidance paper *Making Partnerships Work for Patients, Carers and Service Users* (DoH, 2004g), which was an agreement between government, the NHS and the voluntary sector to strengthen partnerships and improve the quality and range of service planning and provision of non-NHS commissioned services. The government has recently established the 'Third Sector Commissioning Tasks Force' (www.policy hub.gov.uk) to address obstacles to a level playing field for third sector providers in terms of commissioning, procurement and contracting for health services.

All these policy initiatives strongly indicate that the third sector will become an increasingly important provider of services in the future, with government envisioning the sector as an integral partner in the delivery of health services across the UK.

In spite of government rhetoric about the importance of voluntary and community groups' contribution to health care, the sector is currently faced with considerable problems. Although there has been a steady growth in voluntary organisations providing health services, this has not been matched by an improvement in funding structures and in attitudes on the part of commissioners. The sector is still providing services on short-term contracts, with funding not sufficiently meeting the full cost of provision (what is known as 'full cost recovery'). There is a view that voluntary organisations, because of their charitable status, should receive subsidies of their services from other sources. In a recent survey by the Charity Commission only 13 per cent of organisations reported having contracts longer than three years, with over two-thirds of all funding agreements for public service delivery for one year (Charity Commission, 2007), demonstrating that funding in the sector is predominantly short term. The same survey found that 43 per cent of organisations were not achieving full cost recovery for their services, with a further 38 per cent reporting that they only achieved full cost recovery some of the time. In spite of the introduction of the Compact (Home Office, 1998) in 1998 and the setting up of a Comission for the Compact (www.thecompact.org.uk) that is intended to oversee the relationship between government and the voluntary and community sector, there is still some way to go if the sector is to feel confident in working with the NHS and particularly commissioners at the local level. The main concerns are longer term funding agreements, clearer briefs from commissioners, more standardised contracting arrangements and more honest and open relationships between the NHS and the third sector (DoH, 2007f).

A further area of concern is that third sector organisations, in order to achieve a successful partnership with the NHS, are often forced to change the nature of their organisation in order to meet the demands of the statutory sector. A strong element in the partnerships between the statutory and third sector is the aligning of values and culture of partner organisations in pursuit of shared goals. This can mean that when third sector organisations are offered contracts for the delivery of services, the way that these are delivered are heavily dictated by those commissioning the service (Etherington, 1999). A defining feature of third sector organisations is their independence from government and the ability to determine their own futures; this can be severely compromised where a service is dependent on state funding which can dilute the mission and values of a service in order to secure contracts.

This presents a dilemma for third sector organisations which may seek to contract with the state, but at the same time remain truthful to their mission and values.

Examples of third sector health services

Hospice movement

The hospice movement was begun after World War II by Dame Cicely Saunders and has developed such that there are now over 236 hospices in the UK caring for 60,000 people as inpatients, with a further 135,000 in their own homes, making the voluntary sector a lead provider in palliative care. Hospices claim to be unique in their holistic approach to meeting the needs of the whole person, with staff working alongside the person, rather than managing the person, striving to offer freedom from pain in a setting of dignity, peace and calm. In spite of the success of the hospice movement, with its focus on the patient as the centre of care, many hospices face financial difficulty and have no secure long term funding, with the average government contribution to hospices of less than 30 per cent of their total spend (Bennett and Kirk, 2003). Hospices rely significantly on voluntary contributions and legacies and large numbers of unpaid volunteers (www.hospicesinformation.org).

Acute hospital services

Currently, there are a large number of third sector independent acute hospitals, for example, BUPA has 24 hospitals (www.bupa.co.uk) and Nuffield Hospitals has 39 hospitals throughout the UK (www.nuffieldhospitals.org.uk). In the fields of mental health, brain injury and dementia services, the St Andrew's group of hospitals, was founded in 1838 as a specialist mental health service, providing assessment, treatment and rehabilitation services, including short-term acute and long-term secure programmes. It has specialist units providing treatment for adolescents through to older people with mental health problems (www.stah.org). A further example is the Royal Hospital for Neurodisability in London, which provides facilities for the assessment, treatment and care of people who have suffered damage to their brain or nervous system (www.rhn.org.uk).

Care homes with nursing

A significant policy change took place in the NHS in the 1980s with the reduction in long term care of older people, in what were called at that time 'geriatric units'. Much of this care was transferred to private and voluntary sector residential homes for older people who needed long term care. Although the majority of care is provided by the private sector (and is in itself a significant employer of nurses), a number of national and local charities provide care in residential homes where the nursing care is funded by the NHS.

The following websites describe a range of care homes provided by the third sector, including some larger national organisations and smaller local organisations providing services for a specific locality: www.abbeyfield.org.uk; www.bupacarehomes.co.uk; www.jrf.org/housingandcare.org.uk; www.guildcare.org

Mental health services

Rethink is the largest national voluntary provider of mental health services, founded over 30 years ago to give a voice to people with mental illness. They provide a wide range of services, including helplines, advocacy, support, employment, and residential and nursing care. Rethink is partly governed by service users and also campaigns against the stigma of mental illness. It has a set of beliefs which stress that people affected by severe mental illness have the right to be treated with dignity and respect, with equal opportunities in everyday life (www.rethink.org).

Guided Study 9.2

You may have been on placement in an organisation similar to one of those described above or, if not, access one of the third sector organisations websites and answer the following questions.

What is the philosophy and main aims of the organisation?
Are there similarities or differences with the organisation of the NHS?
How might any differences impact on multi-professional work?

Box 9.1   Nursing Partnerships

An example of nurses working with the third sector is community nurses working in partnership with a voluntary (charitable organisation) hospice. For example, community nursing teams can refer directly to the hospice Community Home Care Team whose staff are all clinical nurse specialists. They are able to provide advice on many aspects of palliative care and disease management, including symptom control. They are also able to give information, advice and guidance on palliative care support to the patient and family and carers. This support usually includes home visits which are often carried out as joint visits with the community nursing team and/or the GP. Where appropriate, and if necessary, the hospice team works together with the community nurses, the patient and family in facilitating hospital/hospice admission and discharge. The voluntary service hospice also provides training and education for nursing staff. A strong, supportive relationship between community nursing, the local hospice and the family is essential in the delivery of both palliative and end-of-life care to patients whose chosen place of care is their own home, for example as part of the Hospice to Home service. A further example of multi-professional partnerships in palliative care services is collaboration with health and social care services and the Delivering Choice project with Marie Curie cancer care (www.deliveringchoice.mariecurie.org.uk/about_the_ delivering_choice_programme/)

What do these changes mean to nurses?

Although the NHS has always worked in partnership with other organisations, government policies since the late 1980s have seen a steady growth in the provision of health services by independent providers, whether private health care services or third sector organisations. The range of services has expanded to meet the demands of patients purchasing health through insurance contributions or services provided as

139

part of employment benefits, or through treatment in independent hospitals who provide, for example, elective surgery on contract to the NHS. Many people will have experienced these services. As a consequence third sector organisations have become significant employers of nurses and other health professionals. In terms of the scale of change, research for the Royal College of Nursing (RCN) has estimated that approximately 50,000 nurses are working in the independent sector of health, which includes hospitals and clinics, care homes and hospices, both in the private and third sector (Buchan and Secombe, 2006). Research on nurses working in the independent sector has suggested that they were generally more satisfied with their working conditions, being proud of their organisations and with positive views about their employers and felt their work was valued, in relation to the NHS. They also reported better staffing levels, more manageable workloads and satisfaction with pay levels. There were particularly high levels of satisfaction among nurses surveyed who worked in hospices, where they felt less pressured, were able to provide high standards of care and were positive about their service and felt valued by their employers. Similarly, nurses working in care homes surveyed by the RCN (Ball, 2004; Ball and Pike, 2005), which are predominantly individually owned or part of large national chains, expressed overall job satisfaction, felt their work was valued and did not have to compromise their nursing judgements, although workload pressures and lack of staff were frequently cited frustrations of work in this sector, which is beset by issues of low fee income and a changing ownership due to commercial pressures.

Examples of third sector developments

Central Surrey Health is a new social enterprise, established in October 2006, which provides nursing and therapy services to patients in central Surrey. It is a nurse managed not-for-profit company, that is mutually owned by its 700 staff, who were previously employees of the NHS. It provides services on contract to Elmbridge and mid-Surrey PCT, who fund it with a £20 million contract to provide these services.

Salford Health Matters is a new social enterprise founded by doctors and nurses to provide medical, nursing and therapy services, which is responding to the needs of patients who want more responsive services and those that are closer to their home. It is also intending to extend the range of services available, including hospital after-care, mental health services and counselling services. Its services will be funded by contracts with Salford PCT.

Local Care Direct is a long established social enterprise based in West Yorkshire that provides a wide range of health services including out-of-hours GP services, hospital after-care services and dental services. The service – with a turnover of £17 million – is committed to providing services that are flexible, responsive and innovative, with a strong voice for stakeholders.

NHS Foundation Trusts (Foundation Hospitals) These are a new type of organisation established as independent, not-for-profit public benefit corporations with accountability to their local communities rather than central government control. Foundation hospitals were established as part of a government drive to give high performing hospitals greater autonomy to run their own affairs. They differ from mainstream NHS Trusts in not being managed by the DoH and have greater freedom to decide how they will meet local health care needs. Since the policy was introduced in 2004 over 60 hospitals have achieved foundation status with more applications pending approval. The policy to develop foundation hospitals is not without its critics (Pollock, 2003), who see this new form of organisation sitting between the public and private sector, less accountable, and potentially competing with other hospitals and a further step towards the privatisation of the NHS.

Guided Study 9.3

Working multi-professionally with third sector professionals

You will know from your reading of earlier chapters that there are some essential characteristics for effective multi-professional working. Imagine you are a nurse working as part of your primary health care experience with a charitable organisation for older people. The organisation offers a range of services, including a healthy living scheme where service users can have health care assessments from health care professionals.

As a nursing professional involved in delivering this service, what would you need to know about the organisation and its partners and its service user group before you could provide this service effectively?

What multi-professional skills and knowledge would you require?

You could have included:

Need to know more?

In this text Chapter 1 offers an introduction to characteristics of good multi-professional working.
Chapter 2 explores the role of the nurse with other health care professionals.
Chapter 3 presents strategies and skills for collaborative partnerships in primary care.
Chapter 6 details requirements for person-centred care.

Useful websites

www.ncvo.org.uk
www.acvo.org.uk.co.uk
www.charity-commission.gov.uk
www.dh.gov.uk
www.thecompact. org.uk
www.hm-treasury.gov.uk
www.rcn.org.uk
www.thirdsector
www.hm-treasury.gov.uk

Future developments

You have seen in this chapter that since the late 1990s, government policy has promoted the role of the third sector in developing and delivering better public services, through opening up markets for public services to be provided by new suppliers from the private and third sectors. The third sector is seen to have unique benefits, in its expertise in specialist areas of provision; its ability to connect with groups which are difficult for traditional public sector organisations; and innovation in developing new forms of delivery. This policy is likely to continue into the future, with recent changes in government unlikely to affect the commitment to the growth of the third sector role in the delivery of public services, although it is less likely that large swathes of the NHS will be transferred to third sector organisations in the future, with a more measured and selective approach taken that focuses on areas where the sector's strengths make it a trusted partner of government (Benjamin, 2007). The government continues to see the third sector as a key partner in innovation and design of services, and as a campaigner for change in the way services are delivered, through the creation of an environment that supports the third sector to play an increasingly important role in contributing to improving services. A specific example will be the Office of the Third Sector's encouragement of PCTs to commission and shape services for their local communities and at the same time offering opportunities for the third sector (Cabinet Office, 2007).

Conclusion

In this chapter you have experienced a snapshot of some of the third sector organisations currently delivering health care. The third sector continues to grow as a result of government policy, which is encouraging a greater diversity of provision and at the same time searching for ways of connecting with consumers of health care to improve quality and responsiveness. This has implications for health care professionals who will increasingly be working in partnership with a wider range of third sector organisations in the delivery of services, ranging from large national charities to local voluntary and community groups. Whatever service you find yourself working in in the future it is important that you understand their mission and values and how they differ from the statutory services, as this will enable you to work more effectively across the boundaries of different services, which will each have their own perspectives, approaches and expectations about how health care is delivered. You may find you are working in a context where partner services deliver health care, but also see it as part of their role to speak out and represent the users of their services, and also enable individuals to make their voices heard about their needs and the services that best meet those needs, particularly where people feel marginalised or disadvantaged by mainstream services. The third sector, playing these multiple roles, can help us think differently about services and how they are delivered, and about how the state and the third sector working together as equal partners can improve and bring about lasting change on behalf of users of health care services.

10

Nursing and Multi-professional Leadership
Janet McCray

By reading this chapter you should be able to:

- **define leadership and assess the suitability of specific leadership styles for multi-professional working and teamwork**
- **identify a range of leadership strategies to support the development and growth of a team and its members**
- **review solutions to the challenges that multi-professional leadership present**
- **reflect on the application of these solutions and strategies for your own leadership practice.**

Introduction

In reaching the final part of this book you will already have gained knowledge of a number of critical elements of good practice in a multi-professional context. You may even be applying some of them in practice and in your assessed coursework. Your reading and reflection on the reasons for collaboration will have given you a multitude of messages about team working with other professionals, and also about the need for nurses to be proactive team leaders and players in a continuous culture of change. As you conclude this book, the intention is to focus specifically on the role of the multi-professional team leader. Beginning with definitions of leadership and its form and application in health and social care, the chapter presents a rationale for the current status of some forms of leadership. Ultimately, in order to respond to change, organisations need effective leadership for transformation. The consequences of a lack of attention to what constitutes effective leadership are presented and assessed from an individual, workforce and organisational perspective and you will be drawing on your own experience. Following this the content will begin to consider team leadership and the implications for multi-professional working. You will be supported to think about managing some of the more complex parts, such as conflict, performance management and the process of leading other professionals in the team setting, through participating in a number of guided study activities. These will encourage you to begin to put into practice the knowledge and skills required and help you on your journey to becoming an effective leader, as you end the chapter and this book.

What is leadership?

Leadership is about setting direction, opening up possibilities, helping people achieve, communication and delivering. It is also about behaviour, as what we do as leaders is even more important than what we say. (Sir Nigel Crisp, Improvement Leaders guide, NHS Modernisation Agency, 2005)

The pace of change and the need for organisations to respond proactively to transform rather than reform their services calls for new forms of leadership. Government legislation and its modernisation agenda has set out a different set of messages. To operationalise the NHS plan (DOH, 2000) and to create a permanent shift in organisational culture, leaders and managers at all levels must apply a range of strategies, knowledge and skills to be effective and make it happen; for, as Titchen and Down (2007) write, a strong culture is one where the values espoused are experienced in practice by staff, patients and others.

The substantial transformation of vision, values, practice and models of service explored in this book so far, to achieve a new organisational culture for the NHS and social care requires a move from traditional leadership described as transactional and focused on telling people 'what to do'. No longer do people practise in a single profession team; care planning systems are more involved and service users have a different set of expectations about their role in the care pathway. Performance management means pressure is on all members of teams to deliver and problem solving needs all workers to think and act creatively to gain solutions. Services could not deliver if management practice saw relationships with workers as solely based on a level of exchange determined by what is expected in their capacity at a certain grade, salary or seniority.

Building new services

To create such comprehensive system change, altering entire organisations and how they think and work is not easy or straightforward. In order to build new services, the modernising agendas of the current government, (DoH, 2000) favour a transformational as opposed to transactional leadership style. The massive changes in the NHS mean that investment in transformational leadership, defined by Burns (1978) and cited by Jasper (2005: 7) as a 'process where one or more persons engage with others in such a way that leaders and followers raise one another to higher levels of motivation and morality' is viewed as the way to accelerate progress.

The work of Senge (1990) has also impacted on organisations seeking to modernise. Senge writes that 'in situations of rapid change only those that are flexible, adaptive and productive will excel. For this to happen, organizations need to "discover how to tap people's commitment and capacity to learn at *all* levels"' (Senge, 1990: 4). To create these learning organisations, leaders must be equipped with a number of key skills described as transformational. Researchers Alimo-Metcalfe and Alban-Metcalfe (2005a) offer a UK transformational leadership model, which includes the following characteristics:

Showing and giving concern
Enabling
Being accessible
Encouraging questioning and commentary
Integrity
Networking
Building shared visions
Self development

Creating cultures of learning while developing leadership styles of others

Alimo-Metcalfe and Alban-Metcalfe (2005c) also offer two distinctive transformational leadership types. The distant leader who acts as a role model and inspirer perhaps working at a chief executive level, and the partner leader who is nearby and works directly with you on a regular basis, showing openness, humility and inclusivity. Equally, they do not completely rule out the need for transactional or traditional leadership to manage services and get things done. West (2004: 51) summarises this role neatly: 'traditional leaders tend to be directive rather than facilitative and advice giving rather than advice seeking.' Sometimes following consultation with staff, a decision on a deadline or priority must be made and then transactional leadership may be the best style to adopt. At other times implementing new clinical guidelines may be best managed by seeking advice from all staff involved to achieve agreement on the most efficient response. Gaining evidence on the effective use of resources is most likely to be achieved accurately through a dialogue with staff and also encourage new or unknown insights into a particular situation. Hence transformational leadership should work best here. The key being the effectiveness of the style adapted. Effectiveness is defined by Bennett and Langford (1983: 65) as 'the relationship between achievements assessed against goals and purposes'.

While managerial effectiveness takes into account the organisational situation in which the leadership or management action is taking place, they note the 'Relationship between what a manager or leader achieves (performance) and what he or she is expected to achieve(aims/purposes and goals) within the constraints imposed by the organisation and socio-economic environment' (1983: 65).

As such, complex practice and service delivery requirements require different leadership qualities and solutions. No doubt you have worked with good leaders in your practice. It is likely their effectiveness was gained through holding all or most of the following: good listening skills, a non-judgemental attitude, honesty and openness. A good leader is skilful at giving positive feedback and, where necessary, constructive criticism. A good leader gains trust through doing what they said they would do, while creating learning experiences for all staff and partners in their team.

It is easy to see how leadership could have a very real and long lasting impact on people's attitude, performance and commitment to their service. The style and quality of leadership is also crucial to get results for service users or patients. Morgan (2007), writing about NHS management, observes that 'Independent assessments of the NHS have found that good management makes a vital contribution to high quality health care.' Morgan cites the 2002 Audit Commission report, 'Achieving the NHS Plan', where 'there is good evidence that better managed health care produces better results for patients.' So the impact of bad leadership could be very damaging indeed. Let's consider the impact of poor or bad leadership on your work. It may make you feel unclear about the purpose of work and what it is meant to achieve, making you feel disheartened and unmotivated as your views are not sought. This could prevent you from learning as no feedback is given on your performance.

Poor leadership: impact on your practice

Your practice may not be effective, as you may have no motivation to assess new approaches to care, a consequence being that as your views are not sought you may in turn not seek the views of patients and carers or other professionals about potential changes. You may not be motivated and engaged to change practice and stay up to date.

Poor leadership: consequences for the workplace

These feelings and actions create a demotivated workforce and organisational inertia sets in. Individuals stop feeling engaged with change and possible new roles, while the major resource – the staff – do not work at their best. The workplace becomes backward looking and patient and service user care is less effective if change is prevented.

Having considered the impact and consequences of particular types of leadership in a broad health and social care context, let us now assess the implications of leadership on multi-professional working in teams.

Team working and multi-professional leadership

You know that leadership styles and strategies need to change, so that organisations can enable their workforce to deliver new models of service with a different set of expectations and outcomes. A traditional style of transactional leadership can no longer be the overarching type used to achieve such widescale cultural change. The government seeking to modernise health and social care is educating transformational leaders on its NHS leadership programme, and the General Council for Social Care in conjunction with Skills for Care has revamped its leadership characteristics for the Post Qualifying Higher Specialist or Advanced Award in Social Work. In the third sector the Association of Chief Executives of Voluntary Associations has undertaken research to assess the capacity of current leaders to respond to this different care landscape.

Throughout this book new multi-professional networks, partnerships and teams have been described, all of which have been created to operate and drive this new culture of care. Critical to the effectiveness of these models is the quality of multi-professional teamwork outcomes, which can be make or break for service delivery, underpinned by the quality of leadership in place. In Chapter 1 you examined research on multi-professional leadership roles, and here we look in more detail at team leading skills.

Leading the multi-professional team

West (2004: 54) writes that the 'essence of team leadership is articulating a clear vision'. The leader can then use energy to focus on gaining support, ideas and action from team members to achieve the vision effectively. In the single professional team this process may be quite straightforward but may become less so if professionals from different backgrounds are working together. From your reading so far you will know that different professionals may have different values and views which can also complicate the achievement of a shared vision. Because of this the leader needs to attend to the team's function and how all of its members work together.

Team identity

One of the major challenges of multi-professional team leadership is creating a team identity (West, 2004: 54). During professional education, socialisation through a combination of a series of activities and the ongoing process of learning, results in the development of a particular shared professional identity. For example nurses may feel this when they are fitted for uniforms for the first time, while doctors entering medical school may experience a similar feeling of belonging when they get their basic medical kit, just as social workers in their first module in university explore values in social work practice. This orientation continues as professionals qualify and continue into new roles. Irvine et al. (2002: 311) describe this as an ongoing developmental process for nurses.

Because individuals have become socialised into a professional group identity, creating a team identity can be very challenging for a leader. Changes in professional preparation and more opportunities to work with other professionals during foundation training may gradually make this less problematic, as may the level of confidence of the professionals involved. If professionals are clear about their role, skills and characteristics and that of their fellow team members, they are likely to feel able to work effectively and learn together to create a common multi-professional team identity, despite the very real challenges faced. A transformational leadership style is likely to be most appropriate to support this process, using facilitation skills to engage people in team learning activities. An evaluation of a multi-professional learning project in a primary care trust (PCT) by Allan et al. (2005) showed that to create a multi-professional learning culture in a PCT was very complex, with mixed views of what this involved. Shared aims and values and communication were agreed on as essential to changing the culture, and those participating in shared learning activity spoke positively of the knowledge and understanding gained of the professional roles of their colleagues. As West continues, if a team is to be healthy and grow, then the leader must influence others in the organisation to ensure the team can do its job properly (West, 2004: 55).

Now think about how you might begin to create a team identity.

Guided Study 10.1

You are a clinical nurse lead for a newly established multi-professional team. At an initial meeting you organised a briefing session to introduce the team and the project, where the professionals present seemed slightly disengaged. However, all present agree to a half-day workshop to begin the process of working together. You agree to lead the session and forward an agenda for the morning to everyone. Afterwards, as you begin planning, you reflect on the approach to take.

Ask yourself:

What would be the main goals for the half day?

What sort of activities would you plan for the half day?

How would you determine success?

In completing this exercise you should have considered:

Working towards the main goals of the team

- A review of the team's remit and goals
- The feasibility of these goals
- An exploration of the role of team members

- An exploration of their role in this team
- Planning how the team will work together and setting ground rules for meetings.
  (Source: Adapted from West, 2004: 80)

Activities

- A group work exercise led by a facilitator for the review and feasibility session
- Asking each person to present a short briefing on their role and how they see their role in the team allowing time for questioning and discussion
- A guided activity to explore how the team will work together.

How would you determine success at this stage?

- Participation of all the members with active listening
- Agreement on team remit and goals
- Opportunity to share positives, uncertainty or challenge assumptions about roles
- Early identification of any major barriers to the team remit
- Team development needs highlighted
- A framework for the future team to work within including ground rules and learning activities.
  (Source: Adapted from Hayes, 2005: 189)

Timing is critical in the staging of team development activity. It is clear that initial planning is vital and investment in building and sustaining relationships is integral to success. Attention to the team and its goals should remain part of the leader's role throughout its lifetime, and as in any team working in complex practice situations, there are times when there will be potential for conflict.

Conflict in multi-professional working

The possibility of conflict can be viewed positively. Bernstein (1973: 72) suggests that while conflict has its terrors, it offers magnificent opportunities for growth. Although nurses are often viewed as conflict avoiders (Cavanagh, 1991: 1255). West (2004: 172) suggests that there are three forms of conflict in teams, which he states are conflict about the task (this could be greater if the team is working in a crisis situation), conflict about team processes and interpersonal conflict. You can add to this role conflict (Pranulis et al., 1995: 45) as there can be competing expectations of roles, responsibilities, functions and priority setting for professionals working in a multi-professional team. Loxley (1997: 70) observing conflict in collaborative working, notes the conflict created by limited resources, and power differences among professionals.

What is also known is that the impact of some forms of conflict, such as that which can make us feel uncomfortable and create feelings of confusion can, over time, create emotional problems and physical exhaustion and dissatisfaction (Barber and Iwai, 1996: 111). In turn this could influence the effectiveness of the overall team performance (West, 2004: 172).

Because of the potential consequences of conflict in the multi-professional team setting, leaders and managers need to make careful choices about handling it successfully.

In my research with nurses and social workers exploring multi-professional working (McCray 2003: 170) and resulting in a conceptual framework (McCray, 2005b), the professionals involved had developed a number of leadership strategies for managing conflict. Initially they agreed that there was no right or wrong way to deal with or manage conflict, and that the situation or context will determine the approach. Second, they noted the need to see conflict as part of the bigger picture; for example, asking where in the process of change is the conflict occurring, what political issues may be involved and impacting on the collaboration, and how is power being used?

West (2004: 172) suggests that there are five basic ways for team leaders to deal with conflict and only one is good. First, avoidance, which will only result in the conflict returning later. Next, giving in to one person in the situation and letting them get what they want. This sets a precedent and that person may expect to win every time. Third, competition, which can lead to misplaced energy and resources and the individual who does not win may become resentful. Compromise which may be better but no one gets their needs met, or collaboration which can mean all are happy as all needs are met, and a good outcome to the problem is found. Collaboration means the team should be stronger as a result (West, 2004: 173). Having considered the theory, let us now consider how this might work in practice.

Guided Study 10.2

You are leading a multi-professional review for a person with a learning disability, who is not present at the meeting as she is on holiday. The overall aim of the review process is to agree with the individual and her family appropriate provision of care now she is leaving full-time education. Recently at one of the meetings one of the social care professionals newly involved with the service user had suggested that she might enjoy being in receipt of a direct payments scheme to enable her to choose and plan her individual care. (See Cally Ward's chapter for details of direct payments.) This was met with a very negative response from one of the health care team members at the meeting whose basis for disagreement was that the professional 'Did not know the person'. As the lead at the meeting you asked if the issue of direct payment could be revisited with the service user herself present. This was agreed by all, and one professional agreed to brief and prepare her for the next meeting. On leaving you reflect on the conflict, about its nature and what could be done prior to the next meeting to resolve it effectively.

Source of Conflict

Ask yourself:

What could have been the nature of the conflict in this or a similar type situation?

You could have included:

Confusion about the task that is the overall aim of the review process, perhaps it needed to be made clearer
Interpersonal conflict between the old and new team member
Competing expectations and priority setting in the review process
Status issues in relation to the power accorded to the individuals views.

In the situation discussed, a number of factors could be the cause of conflict, creating a need to consider in more detail how to respond as an effective leader. It is possible that unclear aims for the review caused this situation, or that the aims were not revisited as new members joined the group. However, this seems unlikely as the conflict was about provision of care, a relevant topic for the multi-professional team.

Interpersonal issues are frequently used as an explanation for conflict and if you look at this situation in more detail it could have been the reason for the criticism made. As West (2004: 178) notes when people with different styles of working come together – there may be conflict. West suggests that most of the time people can put irritation and frustration to one side, but if an interpersonal issue becomes a cause of team ineffectiveness then it would need to be dealt with. Here though it seems unlikely that a one-off remark should be viewed as a result of interpersonal conflict. However, confusion over competing expectations and priorities for care could be the cause. Dow and Evans (2005: 69) discuss the challenge of particular professions' views of patient care. Using lung cancer as an example they note that doctors may wish to treat a person with lung cancer when chances of success are low and treatment has side effects. Nurses may feel the results of treatment are so bad that they outweigh any benefits. Meanwhile the person leaves the decision with the doctors. Thus, conflict is present. In our situation related to direct payments, it may well be a professional value issue causing conflict. For example the health care professional may be more concerned that the person's emotional and physical health remain stable, fearing that a move to more responsibility may bring on too much stress for the individual. Yet the social care professional may feel the person would gain from having more choice. Thus the difference in position resulted in a remark made.

Finally, power or status could have added to the disagreement. The criticism made, may have conferred a lesser status on the other professional, of 'not knowing the person': the implication being that as they knew the person better their views should hold higher status.

It takes time to work through the potential cause of conflict in a team, yet ignoring conflict may take even longer. Having come up with the source, it is now time to consider a response.

Guided Study 10.3

Leadership response to conflict

Ask yourself:

First of all consider the leadership style that would work best here.

You could have included:

A transformational style would be more effective here. A transactional style based on telling people what to do, would most likely create more tension, as people would feel less able to express their views to each other or to you, and conflict would go underground,

(Continued)

(Continued)

leading to a lack of honesty in meetings and a subsequent loss of trust across the team membership.

Transformational leadership would involve seeking views, facilitating a meeting to resolve issues and gaining agreement from both parties on the way forward. Key to effective conflict resolution is acknowledging other professionals' views without hostility and working to keep communication channels open (McCray, 2005b: 230).

It is important to think about how you would work to resolve this conflict. One way would be organising a meeting of the two professionals led by you. The focus would be the difference in opinion expressed in relation to direct payments for the service user and seeking to gain some understanding of the different perspectives, before the next review meeting. Your starting point might be asking each professional to share details of their professional role and link with the service user. From this point you can then ask what they feel is the best option for the person and why they disagreed at the meeting. It is likely that both professionals would want the same thing and that should be based on hearing the views of the service user. If difference is expressed you can explore this and draw the discussion towards its basis. Where commonality is present build on it. Your leadership should encourage those involved to seek out solutions to difficulties raised. Throughout, your focus should stay on the service user's need as central.

Using this approach all of those involved gain. The service user view remains paramount. Your leadership has credibility as you did not avoid confronting the issue, and the professionals will have aired their differences and their similarities. Consequently, the team's relationships should be stronger and roles clearer as a result of this process.

Other sources of conflict

Of course it would be impossible, within one chapter, to identity and offer solutions for all possible forms and causes of conflict in the multi-professional team setting. The strategies for conflict management offered here could be used and adapted for alternative situations, although it is important to recognise that other causes of conflict might require different interventions and may need more organisational or individual management as opposed to a team approach.

Leading new services

As you read earlier, moves toward integrated teams and working in new models of service delivery, change the roles and expectations of both leaders and members in team work settings. Good leadership skills can be vital in making sure a team has the ability to deal with conflict, grow and respond to change. This is not just an issue for traditional practices facing transformation, it can also occur in new models of service design when challenges are faced by those committed to different ways of working. In Chapter 8 services to support children and families were explored, and we know that leaders of integrated teams are embarking on new relationships with other disciplines, as they take on the day to day leadership and management of their practice. One example being where social work team leaders may be managing nurses and other professionals in children and young peoples services, working to achieve a set of external government targets. Malin and Morrow (2007: 453) discuss multi-professional working in the Sure Start programme. They observe that 'Imposing externally defined targets on professional working arrangements may have a counterbalancing effect when this affects a professional's capacity to offer discretionary judgement.'

Malin and Morrow (2007: 453) are referring to the impact of a shift in culture that performance targets can create. You will have seen in your practice placements and explored, in Chapter 5, that professionals can no longer work as they wish in terms of determining results for clients or services. Performance targets – such as achieving the 62 day waiting time from referral to diagnosis for new cancer patients and guidelines to support this (DoH, 2006e) – place a series of actions on professionals within cancer services. Performance managers not clinicians may be leading these initiatives.

As the government seeks efficiency, equality and transparency in terms of performance of services to receive results, this may affect some professionals' commitment to multi-professional working. Their own input is less easily attributed (Payne, 2000), with team measures being the link to a range of outcomes for service users. More positively, this should help leaders of multi-professional teams, as everyone should be working to the same targets, leading to less concern about the use and appropriateness of discretionary judgement.

Nevertheless in new services and despite new roles, not all professionals may want to change their practice or believe in the validity of these targets or those managing the processes (Kirkpatrick et al., 2005) and others may require support to develop the skills required.

Leadership strategies to support change in the multi-professional team

In reviewing strategies to support change we return to Senge (1990: 4), for whom the critical success factor in creating and sustaining change is enabling individuals to learn effectively. Having gained the skills and confidence they can respond actively to a constantly changing environment. Many of the team leadership activities set out here begin to establish a framework for multi-professional learning. You may have participated in a multi-professional learning module as part of your pre-registration professional training, or been on a placement in a PCT where a multi-professional learning project has been underway. These may be formally evaluated and assessed, and should have given you an understanding of what forms of activity may be helpful. Some of these projects were referred to in Chapter 1 and here in Chapter 10.

There are a number of other forms of activity which could be established for your team, whose use will be dependent on its structure, size and purpose. The following exercise will guide your thinking.

Guided Study 10.4

You are leading a team of eight professionals from a range of disciplines in health and education who are implementing a sexual health screening programme for young people. The project is going to run for one year with four of the team members permanently based together for this time, and four participating on a regular sessional basis. In order to achieve the project's aims and targets, ways of working need to change and you as leader must sell a new vision of the service and ensure the team members are equipped with the skills and motivation to change. You have already worked hard on team vision, role and identity which has been positive.

Ask yourself:

What frameworks for staff learning and development would you put in place?

You could have included:

A formal system of personal development planning for each team member linked to organisational strategy and goals
Clinical supervision
Mentorship
Peer supervision
Coaching
Group supervision
Ensuring access to elearning tools, libraries and networks.

(Source: McCray, 2005a)

All or some of these actions would enable individuals to gain formal feedback about their performance, their learning and development needs and space to reflect on their new role and multi-professional relationships in the team. Allan et al. (2005), in their evaluation of multi-professional learning in primary care, found that professionals in the project reviewed noted the importance of having one person to organise and ensure that development activity took place (Allan et al., 2005: 6). As the team leader you may take this on, or it may be more effective to delegate the coordination of activity using coaches, mentors and group facilitators.

Through a combination of all or some of the above learning strategies, you can begin to create a positive multi-professional learning environment which can impact on team culture and output. However, in some situations things don't always go well and some people may not be performing as they should in a team setting.

When things don't go well: managing poor performance

At this point it would be useful to reflect on your own role and behaviour as the team leader. West (2004: 181) considers, does the problem really lie with the 'difficult person' or with you or the other team members? Is it simply that you or the team do not understand the person and his or her role in the team? Are they viewed as different? Good leaders will spend time working through these issues first rather than swiftly judging the individual concerned. If you decide that the problem does lie with the individual, you can work positively with the person in identifying the source of the problem, towards planning a solution and setting up networks of support to ensure action is followed up.

Guided Study 10.5

Staying with the scenario for the guided study above. You have identified a problem with one of the permanent team members who, when working in her new role, displays consistently negative views about the usefulness of working with young people in developing community networks. Her responses about this approach and her new role is draining the team of enthusiasm and energy. You are worried it may begin to have a permanent effect on team performance.

Ask yourself:

As a leader what action would you take?

Good practice points to consider:

Management: before discussion with the person

- Identity the problem area clearly – it's not the person but an area of her work
- Identify objective evidence for giving feedback
- Ensure resources are in place to support changes required before you tackle
- Set a plan with timeframe to agree with person around your commitments
- Be fair! If not just one person look for a team strategy
- Ask yourself: Can you be honest and consistent in the dialogue?
- Have you support of other managers or team members? (Alimo-Metcalfe, and Alban-Metcalfe, 2005b)
- Make a time and date (soon) to meet the person and give an indication of what the purpose of the meeting is. It is easier for people to deal with if they are prepared.

In the situation

- Give clear feedback with examples related to the area of performance, so for example in this case it would not be useful for the person to hear 'you are very negative', this is too vague and judgemental (Barton, 2006)

155

- Show genuine concern but be honest – it's ok to be serious and a transformational leadership style would show authenticity (Barbuto and Barbach, 2006)
- Explain what sort of approach and behaviour you are expecting in the future and what the real consequences of no change are
- Set objectives with the person for change that are achievable, relevant, time limited, and offer support or developmental activity.

It is likely that through effective leadership the consequences of negative practice in the teamwork setting can be reduced. By giving the individual concerned clear feedback they are supported to learn from and through the experience, continuing to grow and develop. Sometimes this may not be sufficient or appropriate and the best route for all concerned is for the person to leave the team. The team can then remain focused on its vision and project aims and the individual can work where they can be more effective.

Conclusion

In this chapter you will have learnt that as views about social and health care change and the nature of collaboration and teamwork is transformed, achieving successful multi-professional practice is dependent on new forms of leadership. Here you have been able to explore some of the perspectives on leadership and its dimensions, linking this to team and organisational development and performance. By taking part in the guided study activities you will have had the opportunity both to confirm your existing knowledge and plan, through reflection on the research presented, your own areas for further development in practice.

Conclusion

During your reading of this book you will have noted the massive changes taking place in service delivery and had the opportunity to assess their impact on your role as a nurse in a multi-professional setting.

New partnerships have been described, as support, treatments and service delivery responses change. Throughout you will have noted similarities and key themes emerging. Notably the service user as partner in the multi-professional landscape of care, while the third sector is becoming an increasingly significant partner with the NHS. You have read that professionals will require new skills and experience particularly in multi-professional leadership of professionals from other disciplines, and will be expected to continue to deliver high quality care with constantly limited resources.

Further, while old tensions – such as those between doctors and nurses in the NHS – may be diminishing, new potential areas of conflict and uncertainty are emerging in a wider health and social care context. One example being the move to individualised care for all service users and carers. As the policy intentions of *Our Health, Our Care, Our Say* (DOH, 2006b) become a reality, and the personalisation of social care increases, who will facilitate and manage multi-professional care processes and where and by whom will these new workers be employed? As you have read, the government is supporting more involvement of the third sector in service delivery and encouraging social entrepreneurship in the provision of health and social care in its new commissioning framework for health and well-being (DOH, 2007d). For nurses such developments provide an opportunity to work in, set up or lead a new type of health and social care service and offer individually tailored care and support. New partnerships and alliances are being created and for nurses the option of getting to know an individual well, providing negotiated, creative, planned point of delivery care for people in their choice of environment will be a strong driver for reallocation to this sector.

Currently, working in a social enterprise remains only one of a range of career choices for nurses to pursue, and the impact of these new models of care on professionals and their role have yet to be fully realised or resolved. As these new models emerge tensions are likely to exist as existing and new provision bid for funding of services. Traditional allegiances and cultures will shift as further transformation and re-engineering of services takes place.

For many professionals this future scenario may seem remote and unlikely. It is of course possible that the growth of the social enterprise and or personalised care sector, may remain only a small part of a health and social care portfolio designed to offer a range of options for all in a diverse society. But one thing is certain. As the care environment shifts to include these new service designs, multi-professional working will be central and essential to creating and sustaining partnerships formed through these changes. Where professionals are involved in care delivery they will require advanced professional skill and leadership knowledge with the service user or patient at the centre. As a nurse preparing for this new era I hope that the foundation studies offered here have helped you gain some of the knowledge and skills necessary to further your multi-professional practice and facilitate your future success and effectiveness in this new world of practice.

References

ACEVO (2004) *Replacing the State, The Case for Third Sector Public Service Delivery*, London: ACEVO.

Allan, H., Bryan, K., Clawson, L. and Smith, P. (2005) 'Developing an interprofessional learning culture in primary care', *Journal of Interprofessional Care*, 19(5): 452–64.

Alimo-Metcalfe, B. and Alban-Metcalfe, J. (2005a) *The Transformational Leadership Questionnaire (TLQ)*, Leeds: LRDL. www.sdo.lshtm.ac.uk/files/adhoc/conference-2005-alimo-metcalfe.pdf (Accessed August 5 2007).

Alimo-Metcalfe, B. and Alban-Metcalfe, J. (2005b) 'The crucial role of leadership in meeting the challenges of change', *Vision – The Journal of Business Perspective*, 9(2): 27–39.

Alimo-Metcalfe, B. and Alban-Metcalfe, J. (2005c) 'Leadership: time for a new direction?', *Leadership*, 1: 51–71.

Alimo-Metcalfe, B. and Samela, C. (2005) *The impact of leadership on the well being and motivation of staff and admissions to hospitals in CRT.* Lecture Westminster House April 2005. www.sdo.lshtm.ac.uk/files/adhoc/conference-2005-alimo-metcalfe.pdf (Accessed Aug 5 2007).

Appleby, L. (2006) 'Avoidable deaths – five year report of the national confidential inquiry into suicide and homicide by people with mental illness', December 2006, Manchester: University of Manchester.

Arnold, L., Drenkard, K., Ela, S., Goedken, J., Hamilton, C., Harris, C., Holecek, N. and White, M. (2006) 'Strategic positioning for nursing excellence in health systems: insights from chief nursing executives', *Nursing Administration Quarterly* Jan-Mar, 30(1):11–20.

Atwal, A. (2002) 'Nurses perceptions of discharge planning in acute health care: a case study in one British teaching hospital', *Journal of Advanced Nursing*, 39: 450–58.

Atwal, A. and Caldwell, K. (2006) 'Nurses perceptions of multidisciplinary team work in acute health care', *International Journal of Nursing Practice*, 12: 359–65.

Atwal, A. and Caldwell, K. (2002) 'Do multidisciplinary integrated care pathways improve interprofessional collaboration?', *Scandinavian Journal of Caring Sciences*, 16(4): 360–7.

Audit Commission (2002) '"Achieving the NHS Plan." Assessment of current performance, likely future progress and capacity to improve', London: Audit Commission.

Baggott, R. (1988) *Health and Health Care in Britain* (2nd edition), London: Macmillan Press.

Ball, J. (2004) *RCN Care Home Survey 2004, Impact of Low Fees for Care Homes in the UK*, London: Royal College of Nursing.

Ball, J. and Pike, G. (2005) *Nurses in the Independent Sector. Members working in the Independent Sector from the 2001 and 2005 RCN Employment Surveys*, Hove: Employment Research.

Barber, C. and Iwai, M. (1996) 'Role conflict and role ambiguity as predictors of burnout among staff caring for elderly dementia patients', *Journal of Gerontological Social Work*, 26(1/2): 111–16.

Baron, R.A. Byrne, D. (2004) *Social Psychology*, Boston: Allyn and Bacon.

Barr, H., Koppel, I., Reeves, S., Hammick, M. and Freeth, D. (2005) *Effective Interprofessional Education. Argument, Assumption and Evidence*, Oxford: Blackwell Publishing.

Barton, D. (2006) 'Talent accountability', *Leadership Excellence*, 23(2): 13.

Barbuto, J.E. and Barbach, M.E. (2006) 'The emotional intelligence of transformational leaders', *Journal of Social Pyschology*, 146(1): 51–64.

Baskett, P., Steen, P. and Bossaert, L. (2005) European Resuscitation Council Guidelines for Resuscitation 2005 Section 8. The ethics of resuscitation and end-of-life decisions. Resuscitation 67 ISI7I-SI80 doi- 1016.resuscitation 2006.

Benjamin, A. (2007) 'Voluntary sector and the dangers of hype', *Guardian Unlimited*, accessible at www.guardian.co.uk

Bennet, D. and Kirk, S. (2003) *Third Sector Hospices, in ACEVO, Replacing the State. The Case for Third Sector Public Service Delivery*, London: ACEVO.

Bennett, R.D. and Langford, V. (1983) 'Managerial effectiveness', in A.P.O. Williams (ed.), *Using Personnel Research*. Aldershot: Gower Press. pp. 64–80.

Benson, L. and Ducanis, A. (1995) 'Nurses perceptions of their role and role conflicts', *Rehabilitation Nurse*, 20: 204–11.

Berger, J.L. (2006) 'Incorporation of the tidal model into the interdisciplinary plan of care – a program quality improvement project', *Journal of Psychiatric and Mental Health Nursing*, 13: 464–7.

Beringer, A.J., Fletcher, M.E. and Taket, A.R. (2006) 'Rules and resources: a structuration approach to understanding the coordination of children's inpatient health care', *Journal of Advanced Nursing*, 56: 325–35.

Beresford, P. (2005) 'Theory and practice of service user involvement in research: making the connection with public policy and practice', in L. Lowes and I. Hulatt (eds), *Involving Service Users In Health and Social Care Research*, London: Routledge.

Bereford, P. and Croft, S. (1996) 'The politics of participation', in D. Taylor (ed.), *Critical Social Policy: A Reader*. London: Sage.

Beresford, P. and Trevillion, S. (1995) *Developing Skills for Community Care: A Collaborative Approach*, London: Arena.

Bernstein, S. (1973) *Explorations in Group Work: Essays in Theory and Practice*, Boston, MA: Charles River Books.

Biggs, S. (1997) 'Interprofessional collaboration problems and prospects', in J. Ovretveit, P. Mathias and T. Thompson (eds), *Interprofessional Working for Health and Social Care*. London: Macmillan.

Birchall, E. (2005) 'Child protection', in P. Owens, J. Carrier and J. Horder (eds), *Interprofessional Issues in Health and Community Care*, London: Macmillan.

Birchall, J.L. (1997) 'Patient-focused care: anatomy of a failure', *Holistic Nursing Practice*, 11: 17–29.

Bjorkstrom, M., Johansson, I. and Athlin, E. (2006) 'Is the humanistic view of the nurse role still alive – in spite of an academic education?', *Journal of Advanced Nursing*, 54(4): 502–51.

Bleakley, A., Boyden, J., Hobbs, A., Walsh, L. and Allard, J. (2006) 'Improving teamwork climate in operating theatres: the shift from multiprofessionalism to interprofessionalism', *Journal of Interprofessional Care,* 20(5): 461–70.

Blom-Cooper, L. (1985) *A Child in Trust.* London: Borough of Brent.

Brandon, D., Brandon, A. and Brandon, T. (1995) *Advocacy: Power to People With Disabilities,* Birmingham: Venture Press.

British Medical Association, Resuscitation Council (UK) Royal College of Nursing (2007) Decisions relating to cardiopulmonary resuscitation. A joint statement from the British Medical Association, the Resuscitation Council (UK) and the Royal College of Nursing London: BMA October 2007.

Brooks, I. and Brown, R. (2002) 'The role of ritualistic ceremonial in removing barriers between subcultures in the National Health Service', *Journal of Advanced Nursing*, 38(4): 341.

Brown, H. and Cambridge, P. (1995) 'Contracting for change: Making contracts work for people with learning difficulties', in T. Philpot and L. Ward (eds), *Values and Visions: Changing Ideas in Services for People with Learning Difficulties*, London: Butterworth Heinemann. pp. 148–63.

Bubb, S. (2007) 'Transforming Our Public Services Through the Third Sector', HMT Third Sector Review. Accessible at www.acevo.org

Bubb, S. (2003) Introduction in ACEVO, *Replacing the State. The Case for Third Sector Public Service Delivery*, London: ACEVO.

Buchan, J. and Secombe, I. (2006) *From Boom to Bust, The UK Nursing Labour Market Review, 2005/6*, London: Royal College of Nursing.

Burke, D., Evans, M., Cockram, A. and Trauer, T. (2000) 'Educational aims and objectives for working in multidisciplinary teams', *Australasian Psychiatry*, 8: 336–9.

Burns, J. (1978) *Leadership*, London: Harper and Row.

Burton, C. and Gibbon, B. (2005) 'Expanding the role of the stroke nurse: a pragmatic clinical trial', *Journal of Advanced Nursing*, 52(6): 640–50.

Cabinet Office (2007) *The Future Role of the Third Sector in Social and Economic Regeneration*, London: Stationery Office. Accessible at www.cabinetoffice.gov.uk/thirdsector

Caldwell, C.D., Lynch Komaromy, F. (2000) 'Working together to improve record keeping', *Nursing Standard*, 14(47): 37–41.

Care Services Improvement Partnership (2007) 'Working Together to Safeguard Children', www.everychildmatters.gov.uk/socialcare/safeguarding/workingtogether/ accessed 7 November, 2007.

Carlin, J. (2005) *Including Me: Managing Complex Health Needs in Schools and Early Years Settings*, London: Council of Disabled Children, Department of Education and Skills, with Mencap.

Carnaby, S. and Cambridge, P. (2006) *Intimate and Personal Care with People with Learning Disabilities*, London: Jessica Kingsley Publishers.

Carrier, J. and Kendall, I. (1995) 'Professionalism and interprofessionalism in health and community care: some theoretical issues', in P. Owens, J. Carrier and I. Horder (eds), *Interprofessional Issues in Community and Primary Health Care*, Basingstoke: Macmillan.

Carter, J., Brown, S. and Griffin, M. (2007a) 'Prevention in integrated children's services: the impact of sure start on referrals to social services and child protection registrations', *Child Abuse Review*, 16: 17–31.

Carter, K., Kilburn, S. and Featherstone, P. (2007b) 'Cellulitis and treatment: a qualitative study of experiences', *British Journal of Nursing*, 16(6): 22–8.

Carter, K. (2007) in National Collaborating Centre for Acute Care 2007, *Venous Thromboembolism Guideline*, London: Royal College of Surgeons.

Cavanagh, S.J. (1991) 'The conflict management style of staff nurses and managers', *Journal of Advanced Nursing*, 16: 1254–60.

Chapple, A., Rogers A, Macdonal, W. and Sergison, M. (2000) *Primary Health Care Research and Development*, Cambridge: Cambridge University Press.

Chartered Society of Physiotherapy www.csp.org.uk/director/about/thecsp/history.cfm Accessed 17 June, 2007.

Charity Commission (2007) *Stand and Deliver: The Future of Charities Delivering Public Services*, London: Charity Commission.

Colwell Report (1974) Report of the Committee into the Care and Supervision provided in relation to Maria Colwell. London: HMSO.

Coombs, M. and Ersser, S.J. (2004) 'Medical hegemony in decision-making – a barrier to interdisciplinary working in intensive care?', *Journal of Advanced Nursing*, 46(3): 245–52.

Copeland, M.E. (1997) *Wellness Recovery Action Plan*, West Dummerston, VT: Peach Press.

Crisp, N. (2005) Improvement Leaders guide, NHS Modernisation Agency. www.wise. nhs.uk accessed 17 July, 2007.

Crompton, W. (2007) *Justice for William*, Winchester: Waterside Press.

CSCI (Commission for Social Care Inspection) (2006) *The State of Adult Social Care in England 2005–2006*, London: CSCI.

CSCI (Commission for Social Care Inspection) (2005) The State of Social Care in England, London: CSCI. Accessible at www.csci.org.uk

Cunnington, L. (2003) 'Setting up a deep vein thrombosis clinic', *Nursing Standard*, 17(23): 37–8.

Daiski, I. (2004) 'Changing nurses' dis-empowering relationship patterns', *Journal of Advanced Nursing*, 48(1): 43–50.

Dalley, J. and Sim, J. (2001) 'Nurses' perceptions of physiotherapists as rehabilitation team members', *Clinical Rehabilitation*, 5: 380–9.

Davies, K. (1993) 'The crafting of good clients', in J. Swain, V. Finkelstein, S. French and M. Oliver (eds), *Disabling Barriers: Enabling Environments*, London: Open University Press/Sage. pp. 197–200.

Davis, C. (2005) 'No waiting in vein', *Nursing Standard*, 20(11): 22–4.

Dawes, D. and Handscomb, A. (2005) *A Literature Review on Team Leadership*, London: The European Nursing Leadership Foundation.

De Bleser, L., Depreitere, R., Waele, K.D., Vanhaecht, K., Vlayen, J. and Sermeus, W. (2006) 'Defining pathways', *Journal of Nursing Management*, 14(7): 553–63.

Dealey, C., Moss, H., Marshall, J. and Elcoat, D.C. (2007) 'Auditing the impact of implementing the Modern Matron role in an acute teaching trust', *Journal of Nursing Management*, 15(1): 22–33.

Department for Education and Skills (2007) *Aiming High for Disabled Children: Better Support for Families. Runcorn*: Department for Education and Skills Public Communications Unit.

Department for Education and Skills (2006) *Every Child Matters, Setting Up Multi-agency services*, Nottingham: Department for Education and Skills. Also available at www.ecm.gov.uk/multiagencyworking

Department for Education and Skills (2005) *Children's Trusts: Leadership, Co-operation, Planning and Safeguarding*. Nottingham: Department for Education and Skills.

Department for Education and Skills (2004a) The Children Act, London: HMSO.

Department of Education and Skills (2004b) *Every Child Matters*. London: HMSO.

Department for Education and Skills (1999) *Mapping Quality in Children's Services: An Evaluation of Local Responses to the Quality Protects Programme – National Overview Report*, London: The Stationery Office.

Department of Health (2008a) *A High Quality Workforce. NHS Next Stage Review*, Norwich: The Stationery Office.

Department of Health (2008b) *High Quality Care for All. NHS Next Stage Review Final Report*, Norwich: The Stationery Office.

Department of Health (2007a) *Every Child Matters, Change for Children Delivering Services*, www.everychildmatters.gov.uk/strategy/guidance/ accessed 19 August 2007.

Department of Health (2007b) *Making It Happen: Pilots, Early Implementation and Demonstration Sites. Health and Social Care Working in Partnership*, London: The Stationery Office.

Department of Health (2007c) *Modernising Adult Social Care: What's Working?*, London: The Stationery Office.

Department of Health(2007d) *Commissioning Framework for Health and Wellbeing*, London: The Stationery Office.

Department of Health (2007e) *Fairness in Primary Care (FPC) Procurement: NHS Primary Medical Care and Related Services*. www.dh.gov.uk/en/Procurementand proposals/Tenders/Informationaboutprocess/DH_073435 accessed 20 November, 2007.

Department of Health (2007f) *NHS LIFT Guidance*, www.dh.gov.uk/en/Procurement andproposals/Publicprivatepartnership/NHSLIFT/index.htm accessed 20 November, 2007.

Department of Health (2007g) *Mental Health Policy Implementation Guide: Learning and Development Toolkit for the Whole of the Mental Health Workforce across both Health and Social Care*, London: The Stationery Office.

Department of Health (2007h) *Putting People First: A Shared Vision and Commitment to the Transformation of Adult Social Care*, Norwich: The Stationery Office.

Department of Health (2006a) *Caring for People with Long Term Conditions: An Education Framework for Community Matrons and Case Managers*, Nottingham: Department of Health.

Department of Health (2006b) *Our Health, Our Care, Our Say*, London: HMSO.

Department of Health (2006c) *No Excuses, Embrace Partnerships Now*, London: The Stationery Office.

Department of Health (2006d) *Choosing Health: Supporting the Physical Needs of People with Severe Mental Illness – Commissioning Framework*, London: The Stationery Office.

Department of Health (2006e) *Cancer Waiting Targets: A Guide* (Version 5), www.dh.gov.uk/en/Publicationsandstatistics/Publications/PublicationsPolicyAndGu idance/DH_063067 accessed 16 August, 2007.

Department of Health (2006f) *Expert Patient Programme*, London: The Stationery Office.

Department of Health (2006g) *The Care Service Improvement Partnership: Integrated Care Network. Strengthening Service User and Carer Involvement: A Guide for Partnerships*. Discussion Paper, London: The Stationery Office.

Department of Health (2006h) *Our Health, Our Care, Our Say: A New Direction for Community Services*, London: The Stationery Office.

Department of Health (2006i) *A Framework for Creating a Stronger Local Voice in the Development of Health and Social Services*, London: The Stationery Office.

Department of Health (2006j) *From Values to Action: The Chief Nursing Officer's Review of Mental Health Nursing*, London: The Stationery Office.

Department of Health (2006k) *Mental Health Bill*, www.publications.parliament. uk/pa/cm200607/cmbills/107/rs1071906.411–416.html

Department of Health (2005) *Annual Report of the Chief Medical Officer on the State of the Public Health*, London: The Stationery Office.

Department of Health (2004a) *The NHS Knowledge and Skills Framework (NHS KSF) and the Development Review Process* (October 2004), London: The Stationery Office.

Department of Health (2004b) *Agenda For Change: Final Agreement*, London: The Stationery Office HMSO.

Department of Health (2004c) *Modernising Medical Careers*, London: The Stationery Office.

Department of Health (2004d) *Achieving Timely 'Simple' Discharge from Hospital: A Toolkit for the Multidisciplinary Team*, London: HMSO The Stationery Office.

Department of Health (2004e) *Mental Health Policy Implementation Guide: Community Development Workers*, London: The Stationery Office.

Department of Health (2004f) *National Service Frameworks for Children and Families*, London: Department of Health.

Department of Health (2004g) *Making Partnerships Work for Patients, Carers and Service Users, a Strategic Agreement Between the Department of Health, the NHS and the Voluntary and Community Sector*, London: The Stationery Office

Department of Health (2003a) *Direct Payments Guidance*, London: The Stationery Office.

Department of Health (2003b) *Mental Health Policy Implementation Guide: Support, Time and Recovery (STR) Workers*, London: The Stationery Office.

Department of Health (2002a) *Delivering the NHS Plan Next Steps on Investment, Next Steps on Reform*, London: The Stationery Office.

Department of Health (2002b) *Shifting the Balance of Power: The Next Steps*, London: The Stationery Office.

Department of Health (2002c) *Liberating the Talents: Helping Primary Care Trusts and Nurses to Deliver the NHS Plan*, London: The Stationery Office.

Department of Health (2002d) *NSF for Older People – Intermediate Care: Moving Forward*, London: The Stationery Office.

Department of Health (2002e) *Health and Social Care Joint Unit and Change Agent Team, 'Discharge from Hospital: A Good Practice Checklist'*, London: The Stationery Office.

Department of Health (2002f) *Mental Health Policy Implementation Guide: Adult Acute Inpatient Care Provision*, London: The Stationery Office.

Department of Health (2002g) *Mental Health Policy Implementation Guide: Community Mental Health Teams*, London: Department of Health.

Department of Health (2002h) *Mental Health Policy Implementation Guide: Dual Diagnosis Good Practice Guide*, London: The Stationery Office.

Department of Health (2002i) *National Minimum Standards for General Adult Services in Psychiatric Intensive Care Units (PICU) and Low Secure Environments*, London: The Stationery Office.

Department of Health (2001a) *Shifting the Balance of Power: The Devolution of Functions to PCTs, the Role of Mental Health NSF Local Implementation Teams and the Impact on Mental Health Services*, London: The Stationery Office.

Department of Health (2001b) *The Mental Health Policy Implementation Guide*, London: The Stationery Office.

Department of Health (2001c) *National Service Framework for Older People*, London: The Stationery Office.

Department of Health (2001d) *Valuing People: A New Strategy for Learning Disability for the 21st Century*, London: The Stationery Office.

Department of Health (2001e) *Family Matters: Counting Families In*, London: The Stationery Office.

Department of Health (2000) *The NHS Plan. A Plan for Investment a Plan for Reform*, London: The Stationery Office.

Department of Health (1999a) *Modernising Health and Social Services: National Policy Guidance*, London: The Stationery Office.

Department of Health (1999b) *Modernising Health and Social Service: Developing the Workforce*, London: The Stationery Office.

Department of Health (1999c) *A National Service Framework for Mental Health: Modern Standards and Service Models*, London: The Stationery Office.

Department of Health (1999d) *Code of Practice to the Mental Health Act 1983* (revised 1999), London: The Stationery Office.

Department of Health (1997) *The New NHS*, London: The Stationery Office.

Department of Health (1992a) *The Health of the Nation: a Strategy for Health in England*, London: HMSO.

Department of Health (1992b) *Medicinal Products: Prescription by Nurses Act*, London: HMSO.

Department of Health (1991) *The Children Act 1989. An Introductory Guide for the NHS*, London: HMSO.

Department of Health (1990a) *The National Health Service and Community Care Act*, London: HMSO.

Department of Health (1990b) *The Care Programme Approach*, London: HMSO.

Department of Health (1989a) *The Children Act*, London: HMSO.

Department of Health (1989b) *Working for Patients*, (Cm 555) London: HMSO.

Department of Health (1976) *Fit for the Future* (The Court Report), London: HMSO.

Department of Health and British Institute of Human Rights (2007) *Human Rights in Health Care: A Framework for Local Action*, London: The Stationery Office.

Department of Health/CSIP (2007) *Getting to Grips with the Money*, London: The Stationery Office.

Department of Health and Social Security (1986) *Neighbourhood Nursing – A Focus for Care. Report of the Community Nursing Review. Cumberlege Report*, London: HMSO.

Department of Health and Social Security (1973) *Report of the Tunbridge Wells Study Group*, London: HMSO.

Disability Rights Commission (2006) *Equal Treatment Investigation*, London: DRC.

Doherty, W.J. (1995) 'The ways and levels of collaboration', *Family Systems Medicine*, 13: 275–81.

Dow, L. and Evans, N. (2005) 'Medicine', in G. Barrett, D. Sellman, and J. Thomas (eds), *Interprofessional Working in Health and Social Care. Professional Perspectives*, Basingstoke: Palgrave.

Duffy, S. (2003) *Keys to Citizenship: A Guide to Getting Good Support Services for People with Learning Difficulties*, London: Paradigm.

Dyer, P. and Temple, M. (2007) 'Doctors, discharge and the interface with the multidisciplinary team', in L. Lees (ed.), *Nurse Facilitated Hospital Discharge*, Keswick: MK publishing. pp. 97–114.

Ellis, D., Jackson, S. and Stevenson, C. (2005) 'A concept analysis of nursing support', in J. Cutcliff and H. McKenna (eds), *The Essential Concepts of Nursing*, Edinburgh: Elsevier Churchill Livingstone.

Etherington, S. (1999) 'Keys to success in the Third Way', *Health Care Today*, April–May, p. 16.

Evans, K. (2002) Personal Development Planning, London: Standing Committee for Nurses, Midwives and Health Visitors/Nursing Standard.

Fahey, S. (2007) 'Developing a nursing service for patients with hepatitis C', *Nursing Standard*, 21(43): 35–40.

Freeman, M., Miller, and C. Ross, N. (2000) 'The impact of individual philosophies of teamwork on multiprofessional practice and the implications for education', *Journal of Interprofessional Care*, 14(3): 237–47.

French, S. and Swain, J. (2001) 'The relationship between disabled people and health professionals', in Albrecht, G., Seelman, K. and Bury, M. (eds), *Handbook of Disability Studies*, London: Sage. pp. 734–53.

Friedson, E. (1994) *Professional Powers: A Study of the Institutionalisation of Formal Knowledge*, Chicago: University of Chicago Press.

Gair, G. and Hartery, T. (2001) 'Medical dominance in multidisciplinary teamwork: a case study of discharge decision making in a geriatric assessment unit', *Journal of Nursing Management*, 9: 3–11.

Gates, B. (2006) *Care Planning and Delivery in Intellectual Disability Nursing*, Oxford: Blackwell Publishing.

Gates, B. (2003) *Learning Disabilities: Towards Integration*, London: Churchill Livingstone.

Glendinning, C. and Kemp, P. (2006) *Cash for Care: Policy Changes in the Welfare State*, Bristol: Polity Press.

Griffin, M. and Melby, V. (2006) 'Developing an advanced nurse practitioner service in emergency care: attitudes of nurses and doctors', *Journal of Advanced Nursing*, 56: 292–301.

Guy, E.M. (1986) *Professionals in Organisations: Debunking a Myth*, New York: Praeger.

Handy, J. (1990) *Occupational Health in a Caring Profession*, Aldershot: Avebury.

Hawtin, M., Hughes, G. and Percy-Smith, J. (1994) *Community Profiling: Auditing Social Needs*, Buckingham: Open University Press.

Hayes, L. (2005) 'Leading change in primary and community care', in M.Jasper and M. Jumaa (eds), *Effective Health Care Leadership*, London: Blackwell.

Hean, S., Macleod Clark, J., Adams, K. and Humphris, D. (2006) 'Will opposites attract? Similarities and difference in students' perceptions of the stereotype profiles of other health and social care professional groups', *Journal of Interprofessional Care*, 20(2): 162–81.

Henderson V. (2006) 'The concept of nursing', *Journal of Advanced Nursing*, 53(1): 21–34.

Henderson, V. (1966) *The Nature of Nursing: A Definition and its Implications for Practice, Research, and Education*, New York: Macmillan.

HM Government (2005) *Statutory Guidance on Interagency Cooperation to Improve the Wellbeing of Children: Children's Trusts*, Nottingham: Department of Education and Skills publications.

HM Government (2001) Learning from Bristol: the report of the public inquiry into children's heart surgery at the Bristol Royal Infirmary 1984–1995. Command Paper: CM 5207, London: HMSO.

HM Government (1988) Report of the Committee of Inquiry into the Child Abuse in Cleveland. Cmnd 412. London: HMSO. Bristol Royal Infirmary Inquiry (2001) www.bristol-inquiry.org.uk/final_report/report/sec2chap30_.htm accessed 19 August 2007.

HMSO (1995) The Disability Discrimination Act, London: HMSO.

HM Treasury and the Department for Education and Skills (2007) Aiming High for Disabled Children: Better Support for Families. www.everychildmatters.gov.uk/resources-and-practice/IG00222/ accessed 29 August 2007.

Home Office (2003) CM5730 *The Victoria Climbie Enquiry Report*, London: The Stationery Office.

Home Office (1998) *The Compact on Relations Between Government and the Voluntary and Community Sector*, London: Home Office. Accessible at www.thecompact.org.uk

Hope, R. (2004) The Ten Essential Shared Capabilities: A Framework for the Whole of the Mental Health Workforce, Leeds: NIMHE/SCMH Joint Workforce Support Unit.

Hopkins, A. (2007) *Delivering Public Services, Service Users Experience of the Third Sector*, London: National Consumer Council. Accessible at www.ncc.org.uk

Huby, G., Holt Brook, J., Thompson, A. and Tierney, A. (2007) Capturing the concealed: interprofessional practice and older patients' participation in decision making about discharge after acute hospitalisation', *Journal of Interprofessional Care*, 21(1): 55–67.

Hudson, B. (2007) 'The Sedgfield integrated team', *Journal of Interprofessional Care*, 21(1): 55–67.

Hudson, M. (2004) *Managing Without Profit, The Art of Managing Third Sector Organisations*, London: Directory of Social Change.

Hudson, M. (2002) *Managing Without Profit: The Art of Managing Third-Sector Organisations* (2nd edition), Liverpool: Directory of Social Care.

Iles, V. and Sutherland, K., NCCSDO (2001) *Managing Change in the NHS: Organisational Change*, www.sdo.lshtm.ac.uk accessed 18 Sept 2007.

Irvine, R., Kerridge, L., McPhee, J. and Freeman, S. (2002) 'Interprofessionalism and ethics: consensus or clash of cultures?', *Journal of Interprofessional Care*, 16: 199–210.

Isaacs, W. (1999) *Dialogue and the Art of Thinking Together: A Pioneering Approach to Communicating in Business and Life*, New York: Doubleday.

Jasper, M. (2005) 'The context of health care leadership in Britain today', in M. Jasper and M. Jumaa (eds), *Effective Health Care Leadership*, London: Blackwell.

Jones, A. (2006) 'Multidisciplinary team working: collaboration and conflict', *International Journal of Mental Health Nursing*, 15(1): 19–28.

Jones, A. (2003) 'Changes in practice at the nurse–doctor interface. Using focus groups to explore the perceptions of first level nurses working in an acute care setting', *Journal of Clinical Nursing*, 12: 124–31.

Jones, L.J. (1994) *The Social Context of Health and Health Work*, Basingstoke: Macmillan.

Jumaa, M. (2005) 'Leadership for emotional intelligence', in M. Jasper and M. Jumaa (eds), *Effective HealthCare Leadership*, London: Blackwell.

Kent, P. and Chalmers, Y. (2006) 'A decade on: has the use of integrated care pathways made a difference in Lanarkshire?', *Journal of Nursing Management*, 14(7): 508–20.

Kirk, S. and Glendinning, C. (2004) 'Developing services to support parents caring for a technology-dependent child at home', *Child: Care, Health & Development*, 30(3): 209–18.

Kirk, S., Glenndinning, C. and Callery, P. (2005) 'Parent or nurse? The experience of being a parent of a technology dependent child', *Journal of Advanced Nursing* 51(5): 456–64.

Kirkpatrick, I., Ackroyd, S. and Walker, R. (2005) 'Dismantling the organisational settlement: towards a new public management', in I. Kirkpatrick, S. Ackroyd and R. Walker (eds), *The New Managerialism and Public Service Professions*, Basingstoke: Palgrave Macmillan.

Kitson, A. (2004) 'Drawing out leadership', *Journal of Advanced Nursing*, 48(3): 211.

Kitson, A. (2003) 'A comparative analysis of lay-caring and professional (nursing) caring relationships', *International Journal of Nursing Studies*, 40: 503–10.

Kvarnström, S. and Cedersund, E. (2006) 'Discursive patterns in multiprofessional healthcare teams', *Journal of Advanced Nursing*, 53(2): 244–52.

Kwan, J., Hand, P., Dennis, M. and Sandercock, P. (2004) 'Effects of introducing an integrated care pathway in an acute stroke unit', *Age and Ageing*, 33: 362–7.

Laming, H. (2003) *The Victoria Climbié Inquiry*. London: Stationery Office. www.victoria climbie-inquiry.org.uk/finreport/report.pdf

Leathard, A. (2003) 'Policy overview', in *Interprofessional Collaboration: From Policy to Practice in Health and Social Care*, A. Leathard (ed.), Hove: Brunner-Routledge.

Leathard, A. (1994) *Going Inter-professional. Working together for Health and Welfare*, London: Routledge.

Lees, L. (2007) 'Exploring nurse-facilitated discharge from hospital', in L. Lees (ed.), *Nurse-facilitated Discharge from Hospital*, Keswick: M&K Publishing pp. 3–27.

Lees, L. (2006) 'Emergency care briefing paper: modernising discharge from hospital', *National Electronic Library for Health.*

Lees, L. (2004) 'Making nurse-led discharge work to improve patient care', *Nursing Times*, 100(37): 30–2.

London Borough of Lambeth (1987) '*Whose Child?' The Report of the Panel of Inquiry into the Death of Tyra Henry*, London: London Borough of Lambeth.

Loxley, A. (1997) *Collaboration in Health and Welfare*, London: Jessica Kingsley.

Magrill, D. (2005) *Supporting Older Families: Making A Real Difference*, London: The Mental Health Foundation.

Malin, N. and Morrow, G. (2007) 'Models of interprofessional working within a Sure Start "Trailblazer" programme', *Journal of Interprofessional Care*, 21(4): 445–57.

Manias, E. and Street, A. (2001) 'Nurse–doctor interactions during critical care ward rounds', *Journal of Clinical Nursing*, 10(4): 442–50.

Marie Curie Cancer Care (2008) The Delivering Choice Programme. www.delivering-choice.mariecurie.org.uk/about_the_delivering_choice_programme/ accessed 11 March 2008.

McCallin, A. (2001) 'Interdisciplinary practice – a matter of teamwork: an integrated literature review', *Journal of Clinical Nursing*, 10(4): 419–28.

McCance, T. (2005) 'A concept analysis of caring', in J. Cutcliffe and H. McKenna (eds), *The Essential Concepts of Nursing*, Elsevier: Churchill Livingstone.

McCray, J. (2007a) 'Reflective practice for collaborative working', in T. Scragg and C. Knott, *Reflective Practice in Social Work*. Exeter: Learning Matters.

McCray, J. (2007b) 'Nursing practice in an interprofessional context', in R. Hogston and B. Marjoram (eds), *Foundations of Nursing Practice Leading the Way*, Basingstoke: Palgrave.

McCray, J. (2005a) Read, reflect, and respond. Personal and people development a core dimension of Agenda for Change BMJ Elearning Module Feb 2005.

McCray, J. (2005b) 'Leadership in an interprofessional context: learning from learning disabiity', in M. Jasper and M. Jumaa (eds), *Effective Health Care Leadership*, London: Blackwell.

McCray, J. (2003) Towards a conceptual framework for interprofessonal practice in the field of learning disability. PhD Thesis. Department of Social Work Studies. University of Southampton.

Mental Health Act (2007) http://www.opsi.gov.uk/acts/acts2007/ukpga_20070012_ en.pdf

Mental Health Act (1983) London: HMSO.

Mickan, S. and Rodger, S.A. (2005) 'Effective health care teams', *Journal of Interprofessional Care,* 19(4): 358–70.

Mickan, S. and Rodger, S.A. (2000) 'The organisational context of teamwork: comparing health care and business literature', *Australian Health Review,* 23(1): 362–76.

Miller, C. and Freeman, M. (2003) 'Clinical teamwork: the impact of policy on collaborative practice', in A. Leathard (ed.), *Interprofessional Collaboration: From Policy to Practice in Health and Social Care,* Hove: Brunner-Routledge.

Molyneux, J. (2001) 'Interprofessional teamworking: what makes teams work well?', *Journal of Interprofessional Care,* 15(1): 29–35.

Morgan, S. (2007) NHS Management numbers. www.dh.gov.uk/en/Policyandguidance/ Organisationpolicy/Modernisation/Reducingburdens/NHSmanagementnumbersan dcosts/DH_4113507 Accessed 3 August 2007.

Morris, J. (2006) 'Independent living: the role of the disability movement in the development of government policy', in C. Glendinning and P. Kemp (eds), *Cash for Care: Policy Changes in the Welfare State,* Bristol: Polity Press.

Mrayyan, M. (2004) 'Nurses' autonomy: influences of nurse managers' actions', *Journal of Advanced Nursing,* 45(3): 326–36.

Mullins, L.J. (2007) *Management and Organisational Behaviour,* Basingstoke: Palgave.

NCVO (2006) *UK Voluntary Sector Almanac 2006: The State of the Sector,* NCVO. Accessible at www.ncvo-vol.org.uk

NCVO (2005) *Good Governance: A code for the Voluntary and Community Sector,* www.governancehub.or.uk/GovHub/Content/Documents/Gd-Gov-FINAL.pdf

NHS (2006) *Modernising Medical Careers: The Foundation Programme,* Leeds: NHS publications.

NHS Executive and Social Services Inspectorate (1999) *Effective Care Coordination in Mental Health Services.* Modernising the CPA. A Policy Booklet, London: NHSE and SSI. www.dh.gov.uk/en/Publicationsandstatistics/Publications/PublicationsPolicy AndGuidance/DH_4009221

NHS London (2006) *Independent Inquiry Into the Care and Treatment of John Barrett,* London: NHS London.

National Institute for Health and Clinical Excellence (2007a) *Venous Thromboembolism: Reducing the Risk of Venous Thromboembolism in Inpatients Undergoing Surgery,* London: NICE.

National Institute for Health and Clinical Excellence (2007b) Press Release: NICE Guideline to Reduce Life-threatening Blood Clots in Surgical Patients. www.nice.org. uk/niceMedia/pdf/2007021VTELaunch.pdf

National Insitute for Health and Clinical Excellence (2006) Clinical Guidance 43. Preventing obesity and staying a healthy weight. www.nice.org.uk Accessed 2 December, 2006.

Nolan, P. (1993) *A History of Mental Health Nursing,* London: Chapman and Hall.

Nursing and Midwifery Council (2008) *The Code: Standards of Conduct, Performance and Ethics for Nurses and Midwives.* London: Nursing and Midwifery Council.

Nursing and Midwifery Council (2006) Record Keeping, A-Z Advice Sheet, NMC Professional Advisory Service www.nmc-uk.org/aDisplayDocument.aspx?Document ID=1587

Nursing and Midwifery Council (2004) *The NMC Code of Professional Conduct: Standards for Conduct, Performance and Ethics*, London: Nursing and Midwifery Council.

Odegard, A. (2007) 'Time used on interprofessional collaboration in child mental health care', *Journal of Interprofessional Care*, January 2007, 21(1): 45–55.

Olsson, L.E., Karlsson, J. and Ekman, I. (2007) 'Effects of nursing interventions within an integrated care pathway for patients with hip fracture', *Journal of Advanced Nursing*, 58(2): 116–25.

Oliver, M. (1996) *Understanding Disability: From Theory to Practice*, Basingstoke: Macmillan.

OPSI (2008) Explanatory Memorandum to the Charities (Northern Ireland) Order 2007, accessed at www.opsi.gov.uk 11 March 2008.

Onyett, S. (2003) *Team Working in Mental Health*. Basingstoke: Palgrave.

Orelove, F.P. and Sobsey, D. (1996) *Educating Children with Multiple Disabilities: A Transdisciplinary Approach* (3rd edition), Baltimore: Paul H. Brookes.

Orme, J. Viggian, N. Naidoo, J. and Knight, T. (2007) 'Missed opportunities? Locating health promotion within multidisciplinary public health', *Public Health* 121(6): 414–19.

Orr, J. (1992) 'The community dimension', in K. Luker and J. Orr (eds), *Health Visiting: Towards Community Health Nursing*, Oxford: Blackwell Scientific.

OSCR (2005) Scottish Charities 2005, Edinburgh: Office of the Scottish Charity Regulator. www. oscr.org.uk

Ovretveit, J. (1997) 'How to describe interprofessional working', in J. Ovretveit, P. Mathias and T. Thompson (eds), *Interprofessional Working for Health and Social Care*, Basingstoke: Palgrave Macmillan.

Paciaroni, M., Mazzotta, G., Corea, F., Caso, V., Venti, M., Milia, P., Silvestrelli, G., Palmerini, F., Parnetti, L. and Gallai, V. (2004) 'Dysphagia following stroke', *European Journal of Neurology*, 51: 162–7.

Paul, S. and Peterson, C.Q. (2001) 'Interprofessional collaboration: issues for practice and research', *Occupational Therapy in Health Care*, 15(3/4): 1–12.

Payne, M. (2000) *Teamwork in Multiprofessional Care*. Basingstoke: Macmillan.

Peckham, S. and Exworthy, M. (2003) *Primary Care in the UK: Policy, Organisation and Management*, Basingstoke: Palgrave Macmillan.

Pollard, K., Sellman, D. and Senior, B. (2005) 'The need for interprofessional working', in G. Barrett, D. Sellman and J. Thomas (eds), *Interprofessional Working in Health and Social Care*. Basingstoke: Palgrave.

Pollock, A. (2003) 'Foundation hospitals will kill the NHS', *Guardian Unlimited*. Accessible at www.guardian.co.uk

Pollock, A. and Dunnigan, M. (2000) 'Beds in the NHS', *British Medical Journal*, 320: 461–2.

Pranulis, M.F., Renwanz-Boyle, A., Kontas, A.S. and Hodson, W.L. (1995) 'Identifying nurses vulnerable to role conflict', *International Nursing Review*, 42(2): 45–50.

Public Administration Select Committee (PASC) (2008) *Public Services and the Third Sector: Rhetoric and Reality*, London: The Stationery Office.

Public Administration Select Committee (2007a) Commissioning Public Services from the Third Sector, accessible at www.parliament.uk

Public Administration Select Committee (PASC) (2007b) Press Notice 10, January 24, 2007 session 2006–2007. London: The Stationery Office.

Quality Assurance Agency for Higher Education (2001) Benchmark Statement: Health care programmes, Gloucester: QAA.

Rethink (2007) *Mental Health Carers.* London: Rethink.

Richardson, S. and Asthana, S. (2006) 'Inter-agency information sharing in health and social care services: the role of professional culture', *British Journal of Social Work,* 36: 657–69.

Richman, L., Kubzansky, L., Maselko, J., Kawachi, I., Choo, P. and Bauer, M. (2005) 'Positive emotion and health: going beyond the negative', *Health Psychology,* July, 24(4): 422–9.

Ritchie, J. (1994) The Report of the Inquiry into the Case and Treatment of Christopher Clunis, Clunis Inquiry (Chair: Jean Ritchie QC) London: HMSO.

Rogers, C. (1970) *Encounter Groups,* London: Penguin.

Rose, P., Bell, D., Green, E.S., Davenport, A., Fegan, C., Grech, H., O'Shaughnessy, D. and Voke, J. (2001) 'The outcome of ambulatory DVT management using a multidisciplinary approach', *Clinical and Laboratory Haematology,* 23(5): 301–6.

Russell, P. (2007) *Care Matters: A Guide to the Carers (Equal Opportunities) Act* 2004, Leeds: Nuffield Educational Fund. The Nuffield Foundation.

Sadler, C. (2007) 'Minimising the risks', *Nursing Standard,* 22(4): 24–5.

Sainsbury Centre for Mental Health (2001) *The Capable Practitioner Framework, The Practice Development & Training Section,* London: The Sainsbury Centre for Mental Health.

Sainsbury Centre for Mental Health (2005) *The Care Programme Approach – Back on Track?,* London: The Sainsbury Centre for Mental Health.

Savage, J. and Scott, C. (2004) 'The modern matron: a hybrid management role with implications for continuous quality improvement', *Journal of Nursing Management,* 12(6): 419–26.

Scholes, J. and Vaughan, B. (2002) 'Cross-boundary working: implications for the multiprofessional team', *Journal of Clinical Nursing,* 11: 399–408.

SCIE (Social Care Institute for Excellence) (2007) Research Briefing 20: Choice, Control and Individual Budgets: Emerging Themes, London: SCIE.

SCIE (Social Care Institute for Excellence) (2006) Stakeholder Position Paper 05. Working Together: Carer Participation in England, Wales and Northern Island, London: SCIE.

Senge, P. (2006) The *Fifth Discipline* (2nd edition), Oxford: Oxford University Press.

Senge, P. (1990) *The Fifth Discipline: The Art and Practice of The Learning Organization,* New Jersey: Transworld Publishing.

Sheehan, D., Robertson, L. and Ormond, T. (2007) 'Comparison of language used and patterns of communication in interprofessional and multidisciplinary teams', *Journal of Interprofessional Care,* 21(1): 17–30.

Skills for Health (2007) Mental Health Competence www.skillsforhealth.org.uk/tools/advsearch_results.php?q=mental+health&level%5B%5D=1&level%5B%5D=2&level%5B%5D=3&level%5B%5D=4&adv_search.x=18&adv_search.y=11&page=5&hidden=&selected

Sloper, P. (2004) 'Facilitators and barriers for co-ordinated multi-agency services', *Child: Care, Health and Development*, 30(6): 571–80.

Social Work Scotland Act (1968) Section 12 A. www.scotland.gov.uk/Topics/Health/care/JointFuture/Publications/SWS12A/Q/f Accessed 11 March, 2008.

Spilsbury, K. and Meyer, J. (2001) 'Defining the nursing contribution to patient outcome: lessons from a review of the literature examining nursing outcomes, skill mix and changing roles', *Journal of Clinical Nursing*, 10(1): 3–14

Stark, S., Stronach, I. and Warne, T. (2002) Teamwork in mental health: rhetoric and reality. *Journal of Psychiatric and Mental Health Nursing*, 9: 411–18.

Stroke Association (2007) stroke.org.uk/campaigns/current_campaigns/stroke_is_a_medical_emergency/act_fast.html Accessed June, 2007.

Stone, N. (2006) 'Evaluating interprofessional education: the tautological need for interdisciplinary approaches', *Journal of Interprofessional Care*, 20(3): 260–75.

Sulch, D. and Kalra, L. (2000) 'Integrated pathways in stroke management', *Age and Ageing*, 29: 349–52.

Thompson, A. and Mathias, P. (eds) (1998) *Standards and Learning Disability* (2nd edition), London: Bailliere Tindall.

Thorlby, R. and Turner, P. (2007) *Choice and Equity PCT Survey*. London: King's Fund.

Tinson, S. (1995) 'Assessing health need: a community perspective', in P. Cain, V. Hyde and E. Howkins (eds), *Community Nursing: Dimensions and Dilemmas,* London: Arnold.

Titchen, A. and Down, J. (2007) Mission Possible: How to Achieve Sustainable Culture of Effectiveness, presentation accessed at http://www.wise.nhs.uk/cmsWISE/Cross+Cutting+Themes/ orgdev/development.htm Accessed 17 July, 2007.

Tonkiss, F., Fenton, N. and Passey, A. (1999) *Trust and Civil Society*, Basingstoke: Palgrave McMillan.

Tovey, P. and Adams, J. (2001) 'Primary care as intersecting social worlds', *Social Science and Medicine,* 52: 695–706.

Towle, A. and Godolphin, W. (1999) 'Framework for teaching and learning informed shared decision making', *British Medical Journal*, 319: 766–71.

Training Organisation for Personal Social Services (2000) *Strategies for Quality: Improving Services for People with Learning Disability Through Training,* Leeds: TOPSS.

Tuckman, B.W. (1965) 'Development sequence in small groups', *Psychological Bulletin*, 63(6).

Turnball, J. (2004) *Learning Disability Nursing*, Oxford: Blackwell Science.

Union of the Physically Impaired against Segregation (1976) *Fundamental Principles of Disability*, London: UPIAS.

Unison (2007) Foundation Trust Watch, accessible at www.unison.org.uk/foundation/pages

Unsworth, C., Thomas, S.A. and Greenwood, K.M. (1997) 'Decision polarisation amongst rehabilitation team recommendations concerning discharge housing for stroke patients', *International Journal of Rehabilitation Research*, 20: 51–69.

Wade, S. (2007) 'The nurse's role in facilitating complex discharge', in L. Lees (ed.), *Nurse Facilitated Hospital Discharge*, Keswick: M&K Publishing. pp. 115–47.

Wagner, J., Power, E.J. and Fox, H. (1988) *Technology Dependent Children: Hospital versus Home Care*, USA: Office of Technology Assessment Task Force.

Wall, A. and Owen, B. (2002) *Health Policy* (2nd edition), London: Routledge.

Waller, S.L., Delaney, S. and Strachan, M.W.J. (2007) 'Does an integrated care pathway enhance the management of diabetic ketoacidosis?', *Diabetic Medicine*, 24(4): 359–63.

West, M.A. (2004) *Effective Teamwork*, London: The British Pyschological Society and Blackwell Publishing.

Whittle, C. (2006) 'Care pathways – the future's bright', *Journal of Nursing Management*, 14(7): 503–5.

World Health Organisation (WHO) (1985) *Targets for Health for All: Targets in Support of the European Regional Strategy for Health for All*, Copenhagen: WHO Regional Office for Europe.

World Health Organisation (WHO) (1978) *Alma Ata 1977: Primary Health Care*, Geneva: WHO/UNICEF.

Woodford, H. (2007) *Essential Geriatrics*, Oxford: Radcliffe Publishing.

Woodward, V.A., Webb, C. and Prowse, M. (2006) 'Nurse consultants: organizational influences on role achievement', *Journal of Clinical Nursing*, 15(3): 272–80.

Zarzycka, D. and Slusarska, B. (2007) 'The essence of nursing care: Polish nurses' perspectives', *Journal of Advanced Nursing*, 59(4): 370–8.

Index